GW00702302

# MEDICINE IN EUROPE

# MEDICINE IN EUROPE

*Edited by*

TESSA RICHARDS, MRCP

*Associate editor, British Medical Journal*

Articles from the *British Medical Journal*

Published by the British Medical Journal
Tavistock Square, London WC1H 9JR

First published 1992

**British Library Cataloguing-in-
Publication Data.
A catalogue record for this book is
available from the British Library.**

ISBN 0–7279–0319–5

The following picture sources are acknowledged:

EC Press Office: pages 6, 56.
Sally and Richard Greenhill: page 19.
BMW (GB) Limited: page 26.
Margaret Cooter: page 69.
Gulerie Rudolf, Kliken, Cologne: page 78.
Burnaby's Picture Library: page 126.
Hewlett Packard: page 129.
Ulrike Préuss/Format: page 138.

Typeset by Bedford Typesetters Limited, Bedford
Printed and bound in Great Britain by
Biddles Ltd, Woodbridge Park, Guildford, Surrey

# Contents

# Introduction

Several European countries are currently debating how to restructure their health services and related social services. The debate at the national level is mostly focused on issues such as the government's role in allocating limited resources in the face of growing demand. Internationally, concern is centered on the integration of Europe, the unification of Germany, and the restructuring of the societies in eastern Europe. Interestingly, these three changes are creating similar challenges for governments because they affect both the formulation of health care policy and the provision of services.

In his report, *Perspectives on the Future of Health Care in Europe*, the British health economist Culyer identifies four factors as "mighty rivers of change" affecting health care: the changing attitude towards the government's role in health; the demographic changes, which are causing a substantial rise in demand for health care services; the rapid development of medical technology; and the changing sociological and political climate in Europe. I should like to add three more factors.

Firstly, unemployment, which, although partly caused by ill health, may itself be a cause of sickness. Those setting policies on unemployment and the labour market must take account of their likely effect on health.

Secondly, increasing awareness of the importance of health promotion and protection. Promoting healthier life styles has become an important health policy instrument, especially when the potential costs and benefits of different policy measures are taken into account.

Thirdly, social inequalities. Closely linked with the prevention debate, the consequences of social inequalities are attracting renewed attention. Recent studies in the Netherlands and elsewhere have concluded that on average lower income groups are less healthy than high income groups.

In addition to these factors there are several "internal" changes taking place in the health care sector which are influencing health policy agenda. Foremost among these is the widespread recognition that the nineteenth century model of institutionalised care for elderly, mentally handicapped, and chronically ill people is obsolete. Smaller scale facilities that enable people to integrate into society are now called for. In the Netherlands the fastest growing segment of health care in the past six years has been the provision of small units for mentally handicapped people. Both the consumers and the providers have collaborated in changing the model of care. Old divisions between hospitals, homes for the elderly, mental institutions, home care organisations, etc, are being lost and new forms of collaboration between different subsectors set up—these reflect not only consumers' preferences but also the need for greater efficiency.

Also affecting the policy agenda is the changing position of the patient. Traditionally, legislation has focused on protecting the rights of the individual patient. The rapid development of medical technology that can prolong life has increased the need for new legislation, as has the increased number of people in need of long term care. Legislation should protect patients' rights without patronising them, allowing them to express their own preferences and desires.

Ethical questions regarding issues such as genetic engineering and new fertility techniques call for increased legislation, despite the trend to deregulate power and to lessen the direct government intervention in many health care issues.

Another necessary change in health care is the reassessment of the role of the medical profession. Medical technology is showing the limits of medical solutions, and to a large and increasing degree health care is becoming a services sector in which several types of professionals—social workers, nurses, and different types of therapists—work together on an equal footing.

My final example of an internal change in health care is the search for efficiency. A new generation of modern managers has emerged who, faced with a scarcity of available resources, are more aware of the necessity of efficiency and effectiveness of the devices rendered.

It is not easy to draw any universal conclusions from the changes described above, I will not try to do so anymore than neither do the articles in this book. Focusing on a wide variety of health issues in Europe, the book is informative and forward looking. It is inspiring and helpful to all of us trying to design policies that promote and safeguard access to high quality health care for all.

HANS J SIMONS
*Deputy Minister of Welfare,*
*Health, and Cultural*
*Affairs of the Netherlands*

# 1992 and all that

TESSA RICHARDS

**Although 31 December 1992 is, to quote Lord Cockfield, "more of a milestone than a finishing post," the (incorrect) idea persists that something dramatic will happen as the clock strikes midnight.**

The Maastricht summit focused public attention on the future of Europe. It also sharpened awareness of the power of the European Community's institutions which, providing national governments ratify the Maastricht treaty, will increase from January 1993. General interest apart, should doctors be concerned? How might these changes and the run up to 31 December 1992, with its Orwellian overtones, affect their working practice?

The articles in this book attempt to address these questions by looking at existing European Community legislation and speculating on the likely effect of what is proposed. The articles emphasise that despite a scant legal basis many decisions which affect health have been made at community level over the past decade or so (box). And now that, post-Maastricht, the European Commission is to have a formal health competence, it is likely that more and more decisions will be made in Brussels. Topics covered include medical manpower and training, the price and control of pharmaceuticals, tobacco, alcohol and drug misuse, nutrition, research, nursing, and ethical and medicolegal issues. Introductory articles give an overview of the community's institutions, how health matters are currently dealt with, medical representation in Europe, and contrasts between European health systems and patterns of disease.

## Setting the scene

The inclusion of a "Sante publique" clause in the Maastricht treaty on political union marks an important turning point. For the first time

## Overview of some established and draft EC legislation affecting health

*Mutual recognition of diplomas*—Doctors' directive established in 1975; nurses' 1977; dentists', vets', midwives' 1980; pharmacists' 1980. Directive on vocational training for GPs (1986): minimum two years' training. Future agenda: harmonising specialist training.

*Reciprocal arrangements for acute medical care*—E111 form. European Council has adopted a recommendation for a European emergency health card.

*Pharmaceuticals*—Directives on assessing safety and efficacy of drugs (and medical equipment). Recommendations on clinical trial procedures. Draft directives on distribution, advertising, and packet leaflets. Proposed European Medicines Agency (to be set up by 1993). Some moves to iron out drug price differentials.

*Food*—Directives on additives, food irradiation, radionuclide limits (post-Chernobyl) and growth promoters in meat. Proposed legislation on standards of food hygiene and labelling foodstuff nutrient values.

*Environment*—Directives on air pollution and water quality. Draft directives on exposure to chemical products, lead, cadmium, pesticides, etc. The framework of a European Environmental Agency has been agreed.

*Health and safety*—Directives on safety in the workplace; personal protective equipment; manual handling of loads; use of display screens (VDUs); exposure to hazardous chemicals, asbestos, and biological agents. Draft directives on protection of pregnant workers and young people.

*Consumer protection*—Draft directives on the liability of suppliers of services; safety of children's toys and equipment. Rapid alert system for "dangerous" consumer products.

*Tobacco*—Directives on tar yield and strengthening the warning labels on tobacco products. Draft directive banning tobacco advertising.

*Health promotion*—Europe against Cancer, Europe against AIDS. Five million ecus allocated (1991) to combat drug misuse. Pending: Europe against Cardiovascular Disease.

*Research*—Medical and health research programme BIOMED 1 (1990-4), budget >130m ecu, split between research on: disease prevention, care, and health systems; major diseases (AIDS, cancer, cardiovascular disease, etc); human genome analysis; biomedical ethics.

the European Community will have a legal base to introduce legislation on health. Ostensibly the scope is limited, primarily to "assure a high level of protection of public health by encouraging cooperation between member states," although this is to include "applying pressure on them to act." In addition, it includes a committment to disease prevention, particularly the "major health scourges." These are not defined but will presumably include cancer and AIDS which are already the subject of EC initiatives. There is also a pledge to tackle drug addiction and cooperate with international organisations concerned with public health (such as the World Health Organisation).

Although the text is scarcely expansive and couched in broad terms, it means that for the first time those concerned with health have a platform; that decisions on health can be divorced from considerations of trade and commerce. This is a major step forward, for until now most of the directives (binding EC laws) that have had an impact on health have been framed by ministers of trade or agriculture, serving their own powerful lobbies, with little or no input from health ministers.

On the negative side, there is concern about the potential such a mandate may provide for future legislation. Can we be sure that legislation on disease prevention, for example, will not spill over into health provision? Few relish the idea of Brussels bureaucrats interfering with the way member states run their health services.

Yet EC "interference" in national affairs is becoming a way of life, as illustrated by the British prime minister's protestations when the EC environment commissioner demanded that work cease on British transport projects.[1] As regularly as the draft directives (box) emerge from the Brussels machinery, apoplectic responses follow, pointing to the flaws and inconsistencies of what is proposed.[2] Directives affecting doctors are no exception. For example, the draft directive on the liability of suppliers of services could—unless, as is predicted, the medical sector is excluded—precipitate an avalanche of litigation.[3] A second directive, on data protection, threatens the existence of

---

**European Community laws and other measures**

**Regulations:** laws that are binding, overrides national law, and applies to all member states.
**Directives:** laws that are binding and lay down compulsory objectives, but member states are left to translate them into national legislation.
**Decisions:** laws binding only on those member states, companies, or individuals to whom they are addressed.
**Opinions** and **Recommendations:** statements, not laws, that are not binding.

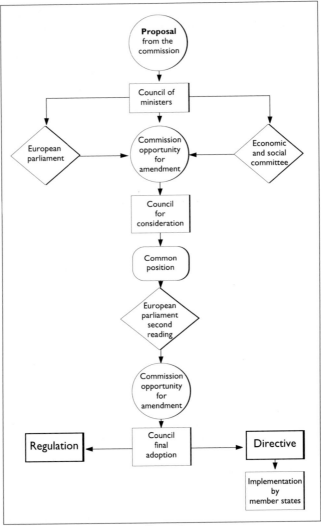

The EC legislative process: one illustration

disease registers and hence much epidemiological research and could sabotage fundraising by charitable organisations.[45] A third, on the safety precautions needed for work with visual display units, has been described as a social albatross around member states' necks.[6]

On a more positive note, EC legislation relating to the quality of water has been welcome, as is the proposed ban on all tobacco advertising. Employment draft directives concerning maximum working hours and the rights of pregnant women[7][8] have been greeted with both enthusiasm and dismay by doctors, for the repercussions on the health service are potentially large. But good or bad the flow of legislation from Brussels, including legislation on health, seems set to increase and it is therefore important to know how it is shaped (figure). The rest of this chapter focuses on this process by outlining the key European institutions and how they were established.

## A little history

There is nothing new about the concept of a European identity, nor about a European system of government. Such ideas date back to mediaeval times, but it was only after the second world war that the desire for union and peace overwhelmed centuries of national power struggles. In a move designed to ensure that Germany, with its massive iron and coal industries, would never dominate Europe again the French put forward a plan to unite these industries across national boundaries. This resulted in the Treaty of Paris, signed in 1951 to create the European Coal and Steel Community. Its aim was to place steel and coal production under a common supranational authority embracing the interests of Belgium, France, West Germany, Netherlands, Italy, and Luxemburg.

Over the next few years moves toward economic unity led, with the signing of the Treaty of Rome in March 1957, to the formation of the European Economic Community. The European Atomic Energy Community was established concurrently. The three institutions were formally merged in 1967 to become the "European Communities." The dominant institution, the European Economic Community, is now commonly referred to as the European Community or EC. In 1973 Britain, along with Denmark and Ireland, joined the EC. Six years later the European Monetary System, linking member states' currencies to a new currency (the ecu), was founded.

In the 1980s Greece, Portugal, and Spain joined the EC, bringing the number of member states up to 12 and the head count to over 325 million citizens. More controversially, Jacques Delors, president of the European Commission, spelt out his vision of the future: a common defence union, monetary union, reform of the EC's institutional

5

structure, and the removal of all obstacles to trade. To this end a draft Treaty of European Union (to replace the Paris and Rome treaties) was drawn up. Despite legendary opposition from Margaret Thatcher an uneasy compromise was eventually reached and the much diluted Single European Act was signed in December 1985.

The treaty was ratified by every national parliament in 1986; its central commitment was to "the progressive establishment of a free market, in goods, persons, services and capital over a period expiring on December 31 1992." It also gave the EC formal powers to lay down policy to this end and to propose (and enact) legislation relevant to its commitment to improve the environment, encourage technological research and development, and, under social affairs, attempt to smooth out some of the disparities between richer and poorer member states. Specific articles in the treaty have enabled issues of environmental and public health and health and safety at work to be considered.

## The institutional maze

The task of achieving the aims of the EC rests with four institutions: the European Parliament, the Council of Ministers, the European

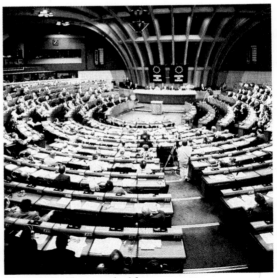

European Parliament poised for more powers

Commission, and the European Court of Justice. The European Parliament holds sessions in Strasburg, its committees meet in Brussels, and its secretariat is in Luxemburg. The Council of Ministers meets in Brussels and Luxemburg. Although largely based in Brussels, some of the European Commission's administrative staff are in Luxemburg, as is the Court of Justice. This institutional maze, which reflects the EC's history and the reluctance of the governments of certain member states to yield their power bases, not infrequently leads to administrative chaos. It also throws considerable strain on EC officials; the image of the fraught (predominantly male), leather handbag toting, peripatetic eurocrat is a reality.

*The European Parliament*

Set up in 1979, the European Parliament initially had little more than an advisory role. Its power was strengthened by the Single European Act, and it is now able to amend EC legislation and to approve some of the EC's expenditure, although it has no influence over farm support. Its 518 members, elected every five years, take their seats on the basis of political groups rather than nationalities.

One of the key issues in the Maastricht Treaty was the proposal to give the European Parliament more power and responsibilities which (assuming all member states ratify the treaty) will take effect from January 1993. In essence it will mean that the parliament will have more say on the EC budget and be able to amend and veto laws on the single market, education, training, consumer rights, health and the arts. Similarly, on the basis of majority voting, it will be able to block EC research and environmental programmes. Importantly, it will also have to be consulted on who heads the European Commission and must approve the choice of a new team of commissioners. Changes which should go a long way towards overcoming the current democratic deficit (for which read lack of openness and accountability) within the Brussels institutions, especially the commission. The parliament has its critics, though: "... served by a bureaucracy of 3600 officials which costs more than 500m ecus a year to run. Efficacy is sapped by rivalries of nationality and party politics ... the cost of duplicating or triplicating some jobs and offices ... working in nine languages . . . all adds to confusion and expense."[9] Furthermore, absenteeism among MEPs is rife and continued wrangling over where and how the parliament should conduct its affairs, counter-productive.

## The Council of Ministers

The council represents the governments of the 12 member states and its key role is to examine the draft legislation drawn up by the commission and to amend, accept, or reject it. Council meetings take place in Brussels and Luxemburg (behind closed doors), participants changing according to the subject under discussion. Health ministers have been meeting twice a year only since 1986; they have come up against the problem that until recently their dossiers have been dealt with by other ministers. For example, the EC's response to bovine spongiform encephalopathy and its risk to human health was shaped by agricultural ministers—and these ministers, together with those responsible for trade and industry, have dealt with much of the legislation related to pharmaceuticals, tobacco products, and food. With powerful lobbies, the interests of industry have usually pre-vailed over health interests.

Twice a year the heads of state and government meet at a European summit to take fundamental decisions about the future of the EC. Before the Single European Act a directive could become law only if it had been passed unanimously by council. Since then qualified majority voting (not one member one vote, but a specially weighted formula) has been possible for legislation related to the internal market.

Council is chaired by each member state in turn for periods of six months. The United Kingdom takes over the presidency from the Portuguese in July 1992 until December 1992 (the last six months before the formal implementation of the single market). The importance of holding the presidency lies in the fact that the country concerned can decide what the agenda will be in response to both the commission's initiatives and its own priorities.

## The European Commission

The commission is the most powerful of the EC institutions. It originates draft legislation to put before the council and parliament and implements the resulting directives, and it can issue regulations on its own accord. By close "participation" in the shaping of legis-lation as it passes through the other EC institutions it has a finger on the legislative pulse at all stages. It manages the funds and common

8

policies that account for most of the EC budget, and through the European Court of Justice the commission can take legal action against member states that fail to implement European law.

Despite its formidable role the commission has fewer than 15 000 staff, and of these a third are translators and interpreters. Furthermore, its key figures, including the 17 commissioners (the "big" countries—France, Germany, Britain, Italy, and Spain—have two each) are appointed, not elected, by member state governments. Each commissioner holds one or more portfolios, which they keep for four years. (The two British commissioners, Leon Brittan and Bruce Millan, are responsible for competition and regional development funds, respectively.) The commissioner who currently holds most responsibility for health matters is Vasso Papendreou, the Greek commissioner: her portfolio consists of employment, industrial relations, and social affairs.

Each commissioner has a small personal staff, or cabinet, which works in (often uneasy) parallel with the commission's permanent civil servants. They work in 23 different departments, known as directorates general or DGs, under director generals who head their own hierarchy of staff. Although a few of these directorates are overstaffed, most—including some of those concerned with health—are run on a shoestring with insufficient staff to deal with burgeoning workloads. Whether the *Economist's* view that the Berlaymont is badly run and its staff deeply unsettled is justified is a moot point,[10] but when I visited Brussels in June 1991 the corridor talk was dominated by how the staff were going to organise, and deal with the repercussions of, a strike.

### The Court of Justice

The European Court of Justice is in Luxemburg and its judiciary is drawn from all member states. European law takes precedence over national law, as the controversy over British fishing rights illustrated.[11] Cases can be brought by individuals, companies, governments, and the commission. The court's workload is immense, and the time taken to produce a judgment is often long. Many countries including Britain are failing to implement an appreciable proportion of established European law; only 37 of the 126 single market laws have been passed by all member states.[12]

### Economic and Social Committee

Another institution with input in the legislative process is the

Economic and Social Committee. This consultative body represents employers, trade unions, and other interested groups; it has comparatively little power.

## Fragmentation of the health bureaucracy

Anyone attempting to understand how health issues are dealt with in Brussels, to get their views across to the commission staff who are shaping draft legislation, and follow the passage of the legislation through the EC institutions must be prepared for frustration. There is no commissioner for health and no one department deals with health issues, so they may have to run the gauntlet of officials in directorates dotted all over Brussels and Luxemburg (box). This is difficult enough from a base in Brussels, but immeasurably more so from a distance. Furthermore, as national medical associations, departments of health, and others have learnt to their cost, protestations from single member states carry little weight with the commission.[13]

---

**Departments in the European Commission concerned with health**

| | |
|---|---|
| DG I: | External relations (Latin America, cocaine, etc) |
| DG III: | Mutual recognition of diplomas, including doctors, nurses, etc |
| | Pharmaceuticals |
| | Food |
| | Medical equipment |
| | Standardisation |
| DG V: | Health and safety |
| | Public health |
| | Europe against Cancer |
| | Europe against AIDS |
| | Nutrition |
| DG VI: | Nutrition |
| | Pesticides |
| | Veterinary medicine |
| DG VIII: | Health in developing countries |
| DG XI: | Environment |
| | Consumer protection |
| DG XII: | Medical health research |
| | Biotechnology |
| DG XIII: | Advanced informatics in medicine |
| CPC: | Consumer affairs |

---

The combination of administrative fragmentation, inadequate communication between directorates, and understaffing—coupled with a noticeable shortage of high calibre, suitably trained and experienced staff—has not been a good recipe for legislative vision. And with no set brief, small wonder that the EC's approach to shaping health policy has been criticised as uncoordinated and ineffectual.

## Changes in the offing

The Maastricht Treaty broadened the activities of the EC's 12 member states more than it deepened the powers of its institutions. It also endorsed the "three pillar concept" which envisages the European Council "sitting astride" three entities known collectively as the European Union. One pillar will be the old EC probably with single currency responsibilities, the second will be concerned with foreign and security policy, the third with internal security—immigration, asylum, and policing.[14]

By pitching for a huge increase in the EC's resources, largely to pay for the promises pledged at Maastricht, Mr Delors has initiated a heated Euro debate.[15] This is being accompanied by an equally crucial debate on how the EC institutions will have to adapt to cope with the expansion of the community to 20 or more members.[16]

## Conclusion

Although the EC has now acquired a formal competence for health, its failure to appoint a commissioner for health means that access to, and influence on, the various different departments and officials shaping health policy and drafting legislation in Brussels will remain difficult. With the pace of legislation set to increase this is worrying. The promise of more commission staff to cope with the increased workload envisaged in implementing the Maastricht Treaty suggests movement on the health front. Under these circumstances recruiting people of the right calibre and experience will be important. What would help much more, however, would be some internal restructuring so that the commission had a common focus which would take responsibility for coordinating health related activities. In recognition of pending change everyone concerned with health seems to have "woken up to Europe" and the need to get their voices heard in Brussels. There is much talk of the need to fill the health policy vacuum and define which health matters are best tackled at com-

11

munity level and which should remain a matter of national concern. Non-professional and non-governmental organisations have been as active on this front as ministers of health and organisations and associations representing doctors.[17] What has been achieved beyond the rhetoric is hard to gauge, but at least the ball is rolling.

1 Oakley R. Major protests at EC road call. *The Times* 1991 Oct 22:10.
2 Water boiler directive from EC raises temperatures. *Independent* 1991 July 13:6.
3 Liability of suppliers of services. *Euro Brief (BMA)* 1991;no 28:283.
4 Proposal for a council directive concerning the protection of individuals in relation to the processing of personal data. *Official Journal of the European Communities* No C 1989 Nov 5:277/3-12. (90/C 277/03.)
5 Grant G. Data protection and use of mailing lists. *Euronews* 1991 May 5:1.
6 A new sprout from Brussels. *Lancet* 1991;337:1317-8.
7 Organisation of working time. *Euro Brief (BMA)* 1991; no 31:312.
8 Pallot P. EC charter gives mothers to be workplace deal. *Daily Telegraph* 1990 Dec 4:6.
9 European parliament heal thyself. *Economist* 1991 Apr 13:54-5.
10 A view from the Brussels boiler room. *Economist* 1991 June 1:52.
11 EC fishes in troubled waters. *Independent* 1991 July 26:6.
12 Policing Europe's single market: laws unto themselves. *Economist* 1991 June 22:98.
13 Schools brief. My, how you've grown. *Economist* 1992 January 25:55.
14 EC extortion. *The Times* 1992 February 13:13.
15 Big is beautiful. *Economist* 1992 January 11:50.
16 Richards T. Edging into Europe. *BMJ* 1991;302:1173.
17 Scott-Samuel A. A public health alliance for Europe. *BMJ* 1991;303:737-8.

# European health challenges

TONY SMITH

Middle aged men and women in Britain are three times as likely to die from coronary heart disease as their counterparts in France, despite being separated by only a few miles of English Channel. As far as heart disease is concerned (fig 1) Europe is clearly divided into northern and southern belts with very different mortality rates. Breast cancer kills twice as many women in Britain as in Greece. But the French and the other southern Europeans don't live any longer: they die of different diseases such as alcoholic cirrhosis of the liver and from road accidents.

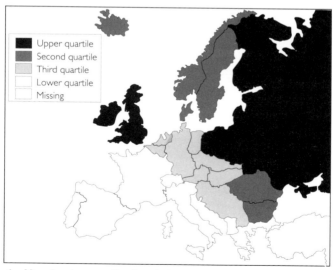

Figure 1—Map showing mortality from ischaemic heart disease in Europe (expressed by quartiles)

These contrasts in health were until recently of interest mainly to epidemiologists, but they are now becoming of wider concern for two main reasons. Firstly, as Britain moves slowly to closer integration into the European Community its citizens are simply becoming more interested in their neighbours—and wanting some of the good things they see over the metaphorical fence. Secondly, the integration process is highlighting the differences between the countries, and their health and health care systems are seen as strikingly varied in a continent that is moving towards a monoculture in finance, television, sport, and politics. Pressure will come increasingly on European countries to bring their health services and the health of their citizens up to at least European average levels. So what are these levels?

## Monitoring health

Monitoring the health of the countries of Europe has been given a substantial impetus by the World Health Organisation's Health for All programme. This global programme as applied to Europe was agreed as a policy in 1984 by the 32 member states of the European region of WHO, which extends from Greenland to the former Soviet Union and the Mediterranean. The programme set 38 targets to be achieved by specific years (1990, 1995, and 2000) by all the countries of the region under five broad headings: equity, morbidity and mortality, lifestyle, environment, and health services, and it introduced indicators to measure movement towards these targets (box).

In practical terms the adoption of this policy means that the health authorities of the 32 nations of Europe have undertaken to collect data ranging from infant and maternal mortality, life expectation, mortality from heart disease and the common cancers, and mortality from road accidents to immunisation rates against infectious diseases, the proportion of dietary energy obtained from fat, and the organisation of primary medical care.

Each of the 32 European countries that agreed the policy also agreed to draw up its own strategy for achieving the goals. This requires each country to record its current standing on each of the measures—from mortality to levels of pollution of the sea and rivers—to set out what actions are needed to achieve the required improvements, and to establish a programme to ensure that the changes are made. The deadline for drawing up the programme was 1990, and most of the 32 have produced health charters of some kind. Britain is one of the laggards; early this year the only part of the United

---

**Selected targets from WHO's Health for All programme**

- Differences in health status between countries and between groups within countries should be reduced by at least 25% by the year 2000 by improving the health of the disadvantaged (target 1)
- The average years people live free from major disease or disability should be increased by at least 10% (target 4)
- There should be no indigenous measles, polio, neonatal tetanus, congenital rubella, diphtheria, congenital syphilis, or malaria in the region by the year 2000 (target 5)
- Mortality from diseases of the circulatory system and from cancer in people under 65 should be cut by at least 15% (targets 9 and 10)
- Clear targets should be set by member states for positive health behaviours such as there being 80% of non-smokers in the adult population and for decreases in damaging behaviour such as overuse of alcohol (targets 16 and 17)
- Clear targets should also be set for making the environment more healthy by achieving safe drinking water for the whole population and by reducing air pollution and the pollution of rivers and seas (targets 18-25)

---

Kingdom to have met the deadline was Wales, which has a clearly set out programme covering all the targets. In midsummer the British government produced its own belated response for England and Scotland. *The Health of the Nation* identified areas for action but proposed further consultation before setting a full range of specific, numerically precise health targets and the dates for achieving them. Health targets have come on to the agenda, but only at the last minute.

## Demographic data

In 1990 the population of Europe was 846 million, and with the exception of Turkey all the nations had reached what demographers term the post-transitional stage, with a low fertility and a low mortality. Nevertheless, by the year 2025 the population is expected to have reached 968 million (fig 2). From the viewpoint of health planners the more important statistic is that between 1990 and 2025 the numbers of people aged over 60 will have risen from 140m to 224m, an increase of 62%. (This figure is not an estimate but a fact— all these 224m people are alive at the present time and their life expectation is known fairly accurately.) Applying existing data about the age related incidence of common diseases to these changes in the

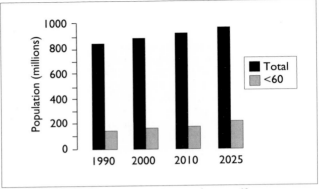

Figure 2—Population of Europe and proportion over 60

age profile of the region shows that there will be a 50% increase in demand for treatment of coronary heart disease and smaller but still substantial increases in the demand for treatment of diabetes and the common cancers. These dramatic increases could, however, be avoided if changes in lifestyle could be achieved sufficient to reduce the incidence of the common diseases by a substantial fraction— ideally by one third.

## Variations in disease

Reducing the incidence of common diseases by one third in 35 years might seem a totally unrealistic objective—except that within Europe the incidence of these diseases already varies to that extent.

Heart disease accounts for 35% of deaths in men and 30% in women aged 25-64, but these are average figures. Age adjusted mortality for ischaemic heart disease in men ranges from 115 in France and 123 in Greece to 223 in western Germany and 355 in the United Kingdom. The western European league leader is Finland, but both Czecho-slovakia (409) and the former Soviet Union (486) have even higher rates (table I). The rates in women are roughly half those in men.

For stroke, by contrast, the northern European countries do rather better: Sweden and Netherlands have an age adjusted mortality for men of around 80, the British figure is 110, and the highest rates (253) are in eastern Europe and Portugal (table II). Similar data are found for women.

Within Europe as a whole mortality from cancer has been increas-

TABLE I—Age adjusted mortality from ischaemic heart disease (1986 data)

| | Men | Women |
|---|---|---|
| France | 115 | 49 |
| Greece | 123 | 50 |
| Italy | 141 | 70 |
| Netherlands | 238 | 99 |
| Germany | 242 | 108 |
| Denmark | 333 | 164 |
| United Kingdom | 355 | 161 |

TABLE II—Age adjusted mortality from stroke (1986 data)

| | Men | Women |
|---|---|---|
| Sweden | 78 | 66 |
| Denmark | 80 | 66 |
| Netherlands | 80 | 64 |
| United Kingdom | 110 | 97 |
| Hungary | 216 | 165 |
| Portugal | 253 | 191 |

ing since 1970, partly as a result of declines in deaths from stroke and heart disease. Total mortality from cancer shows less variation from country to country than mortality from stroke and heart disease, but there are some substantial exceptions. Aged adjusted mortality in women from breast cancer ranges from around 20 in Greece, Portugal, and Spain to around 28 in France and Norway and around 40 in Denmark. Britain has the highest rate in Europe—42 per 100 000 (fig 3). Heart disease and stroke are both substantially preventable by using existing knowledge, and the same is true of at least some cancers. For others mortality can be reduced by screening and early treatment. These are the challenges that need to be met in the coming decades, some progress is being made in changing health related behaviour.

## Smoking and alcohol

In the past 25 years or so the prevalence of smoking has declined in most European countries. The exceptions have been those countries in which there was an initially low rate in women—Austria, Finland, western Germany, Italy, and Norway—in which the numbers of women smoking have risen.

Data on alcohol consumption are collected by the industry and are

17

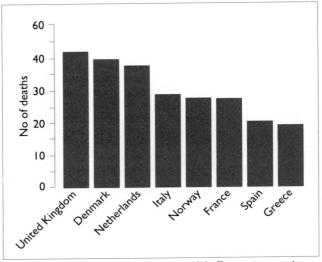

Figure 3—Mortality from breast cancer in eight European countries

given as consumption per person aged over 15. Such data conceal the reality that in many countries around 10% of the population drink half the total amount of alcohol consumed and many adults (up to 50% in some countries) drink no alcohol at all. Between 1980 and 1986 most of the countries with high rates showed some decline, around 10% in most cases. Consumption rose, however, in some countries, including Denmark, Portugal, and Switzerland. Britain is around the midpoint of the European league table.

## Accidents

Improvements in the control of infectious diseases have made accidents the leading cause of death in children and young adults, and road accidents account for around half the total of accidental deaths. Nevertheless during the 1980s overall mortality in Europe from road accidents declined by 18%. Low rates (below 10 per 100 000) were seen in Britain and the Scandinavian countries while relatively high rates (between 15 and 20 per 100 000) were reported from Greece, Belgium, France, Hungary, and Portugal.

Accidents in the home affect mainly the under 5s and the over 70s, in whom falls are the main cause of injury. Accidents at work account

18

for only a fraction of occupational morbidity and mortality, much of which is related to occupational disease.

## Diet

The contribution of variations in national diets to the differences seen in Europe in mortality from diseases such as ischaemic heart disease and breast cancer remains controversial. The main focus of attention in recent years has been on fats, with the northern European countries consuming large amounts of animal and dairy fats, whereas the southern countries use more vegetable fats such as olive oil. The goal set by WHO for fat consumption is that it should contribute between 20% and 30% of the total energy consumption, but it has set an intermediate target of 35%. The current data show that southern European countries such as Turkey and Portugal have low figures while the northern European countries have high consumptions— especially of saturated fats. Nevertheless the picture is not as clear as is sometimes suggested by the health campaigners.

Epidemiologists are struggling to explain those data showing that in all countries with a declining mortality from ischaemic heart disease the total fat consumption has increased in the same time period (with

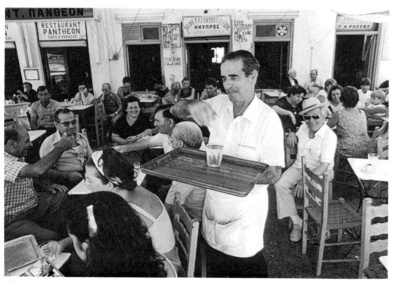

Why are the Greeks so healthy?

19

the exceptions of Britain and Iceland). In many of these countries, however, the increase in fat consumption was relatively greater in vegetable fat, and animal fat consumption actually decreased in Finland, Iceland, Norway, Sweden, and Britain. In those countries in which mortality from ischaemic heart disease was either static or increasing the consumption of total fat and animal fat had also risen (with the exceptions of France and Yugoslavia).

## Life expectancy and happiness

Life expectancy at birth is a crude measure of health, and the whole European region has long since passed the global target of 60 years. Between 1970 and 1985 life expectancy at birth increased by around 2·7 years for the whole region—to around 74 years. The trend is now slowing down, however, as the natural life span is approached. The small scope for further improvement is shown by a calculation: if infant mortality was abolished the resulting increase in life expectancy would be less than one year. Nevertheless there is still a substantial difference in life expectancy between men (70·6 years) and women (77·3 years), much of which is attributable to sex differences in lifestyle (smoking, alcohol, and violent behaviour) and is in theory amenable to change. Differences in life expectancy between countries in Europe are relatively small (fig 4), reflecting the progress that all have made towards achieving a natural lifespan for their citizens. Variations in national cultures have a greater effect on the causes of death than on overall lifespan: the variations within Europe in death rates from individual diseases are still substantial.

Health educators are sometimes confronted with the comment that there is little point in extending the lifespan if the extra years are spent struggling with physical or mental disabilities. Clearly the target should be to prolong the life expectancy free of disability, a measure that has been promoted by WHO as a preferred measure of the outcome of attempts to improve health. Attempts have been made to use this measure in England, France, and the United States. The data suggest that advances in reducing mortality have been accompanied by slower progress in reducing morbidity. People live longer but have to put up with disability for longer, too. Over the 10 years between 1976 and 1985 in England the absolute number of years to be lived with disability increased by 1·3 years in men to 13·1 years and by 2·2 years in women to 16·2 years. Broadly comparable data have been

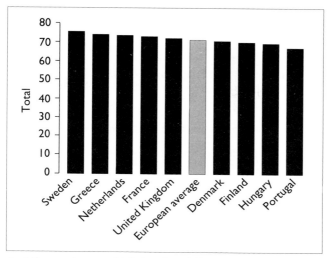

Figure 4—Life expectancy at birth in selected European countries and European average

reported from France, where women may expect to have 11·7 years of disability and men 8·8 years.

This prolongation of disability has been seen by some authorities as a transitional phase. Since the natural lifespan free of disease is limited genetically to around 85 years, improved health should lead to progressive postponement of the onset of degenerative diseases such as arthritis and atherosclerosis, and this should eventually "square off" the morbidity curve until the period of disability becomes only a few months. Whether this optimistic viewpoint is correct will become apparent in the next few years.

## Conclusion

The countries of Europe share the same health problems—a growing number of old people and an ever increasing range of medical interventions from which they can benefit. A substantial increase in demand seems inevitable.

One possible glimmer of hope for the health planners is that the incidence of some of the major diseases might be reducible in those countries with high rates. Mortalities from stroke and heart disease have fallen in many countries as have both mortality and morbidity from road accidents. Full use of epidemiological data may lead to

21

more preventive strategies. Sadly, Britain, as is so often the case, has been dragging along behind the rest of Europe in recognising the need for a health policy and setting targets for the immediate future.

The data in this chapter are taken from statistics collected and analysed by the World Health Organisation Regional Office for Europe and published in two reports:

Van Oyen HJ. *Health for all in Europe: an epidemiological review*. Copenhagen: WHO, 1990.
WHO Regional Office for Europe. *Monitoring of the strategy for health for all by the year 2000. Part 1: the situation in the European region, 1987/88*. Copenhagen: WHO, 1989.
Data are also published by WHO Europe on a diskette: Eurostat (HFA Indicators) Programme.

# European health care systems

TONY SMITH

Every European country is worried about the cost of health care, and most are looking for ways of reorganising their health systems in the hope of reducing costs (see box).

In the 1970s and early 1980s expenditure on health rose faster than the growth in the economy in almost all countries in the Organisation for Economic Cooperation and Development (the OECD includes not only the countries of western Europe but also Japan, the United States, Canada, and Australia). The reasons are familiar enough. Firstly, in all these countries the proportion of old people in the population has been rising, and old people are the main consumers of health care. Secondly, technical and pharmaceutical innovations in health care have led to a real increase in demand for procedures such as joint replacement and for expensive drugs such as erythropoietin. This differential increase in health expenditure is commonly expressed as a ratio, known as the elasticity, between growth in expenditure per citizen on health and the per capita growth in the country's gross domestic product (GDP). Between 1975 and 1987 the average elasticity in OECD countries was 1·1—indicating that health spending was growing at a 10% faster rate than the GDP. The elasticities ranged from 0·9 in Denmark and 1·1 in the United Kingdom to 1·3 in the United States, Belgium, and Japan. Since 1987 economic recession has led to slower growth rates in GDP and the elasticity ratio has widened. In some European countries—Germany and Sweden—expenditure on health has declined in the past three years as a proportion of GDP (see table) while in other countries it has levelled off.

## Current proposals for modification to health care in European countries

Britain is by no means alone in going through a period of rapid change in the system of health care. Most of our European neighbours are looking for ways of making their systems more efficient—or at least for ways of slowing the apparently remorseless rise in costs. Some of these proposals were discussed at a conference in Brussels in June 1991; among the talking points were the following.

France has seen spending on health accelerate far beyond the annual rise in GDP and is looking for ways of reducing its overcapacity. There is talk of cutting the number of general practitioners by 20 000 and of substantial cuts in numbers of hospital beds. As immediate measures public hospitals have been given overall budgets with cash limits and the payments required from patients have been increased. Other proposals include a revised system of reimbursements based on the American concept of diagnosis related groups.

Netherlands attempted in 1988 to introduce a system of regulated competition among insurance companies and among providers of health care. Individual citizens will get a subsidy to help them buy health insurance (which will remain compulsory). The subsidy will come from a central fund dependent on premiums paid by the tax collector. The competing insurance companies will offer different packages of benefits. The target date for the implementation of these proposals was originally set as 1992, but it has now been postponed to 1995.

The Germans are currently most concerned to find ways of integrating the inhabitants of eastern Germany into the existing, very expensive, health care system.

In Greece there has been growing recognition of what is termed the "access trap"—the standards of care provided by many of the sickness funds are inadequate, but the private services are too expensive for most people. Greek health care for most people is based on a black economy in which patients make illegal payments to doctors to top up the doctors' inadequate salaries and reimbursement fees. This black economy is said to amount to 2% of the GDP. According to one speaker at the Brussels conference there is "a labyrinth of institutions, standards, and interests but no plans—only a lot of disillusion."

Spain is making slow progress towards introducing universal coverage through multiple financing; this will be based on a health insurance system that will require substantial contributions from employers.

Health expenditure in selected European countries and United States. Figures are US dollars (percentage of GDP)

|                  | 1970        | 1980        | 1989         |
|------------------|-------------|-------------|--------------|
| Belgium          | 123 (4·1)   | 513 (6·3)   | 980 (7·2)    |
| Denmark          | 209 (6·1)   | 571 (6·8)   | 912 (6·3)    |
| France           | 192 (5·8)   | 656 (7·6)   | 1274 (8·7)   |
| Germany          | 199 (5·9)   | 749 (8·5)   | 1232 (8·2)   |
| Greece           | 62 (4·0)    | 196 (4·3)   | 371 (5·1)    |
| Netherlands      | 207 (6·0)   | 707 (8·2)   | 1135 (8·3)   |
| Sweden           | 274 (7·2)   | 864 (9·5)   | 1361 (8·8)   |
| United Kingdom   | 146 (4·5)   | 454 (5·8)   | 836 (5·8)    |
| United States    | 346 (7·4)   | 1059 (9·3)  | 2354 (11·8)  |

## Basic models

Just as every unhappy family is unhappy in its own way so each country in the OECD has evolved a unique health care system, each of which is unsatisfactory in some respects. The main division between health systems is whether they are funded primarily from taxation (as in Britain, Denmark, Italy, and Sweden) or from some form of social insurance (as in Belgium, France, Germany, Netherlands, and Greece).

Social insurance for health was introduced in Germany under Bismarck, and in those countries which use the system enrolment in an insurance scheme is usually obligatory for all low paid workers. Usually the contributions made by workers cover themselves and their family and vary with income, so that the better paid subsidise the less well paid and the young and single subsidise the elderly and those with large families. In some countries, such as France and Germany, the contributions to the schemes are shared between the employee and the employer: for example, the weekly contribution of car workers in Germany is 6% of their earnings and the employers pay in a further 6% on their behalf.

Higher earners may choose to pay higher premiums into alternative insurance plans that offer wider or more generous benefits. The elderly, the unemployed, and chronic sick are included in the basic insurance schemes, their contributions being paid by the state. In striking contrast with the United States, all countries in the European Economic Community have accepted for many years the principle of provision of health care as a right for the whole population.

In countries with social insurance schemes there may be few or

25

many insurance plans. Often there are a few large non-profit health funds and a larger number of "private," for profit schemes. France has three main sickness funds—for salaried employees, for farmers and agricultural workers, and for the self employed. In Belgium the many mutual aid societies have religious and political affiliations. In theory the existence of multiple schemes encourages competition, but in practice the choice open to an individual worker may be fairly small. Higher paid people do, however, have a wider choice in most countries with insurance based health care.

Insurance based health care is not, however, an example of a free market in health: in all these countries the government exerts some control over the running of the schemes and in most it plays a major part in determining the premiums paid by workers and the fees paid by the schemes to doctors and to hospitals. Typically there is some sort of annual negotiation among all the parties—government, sickness funds, private insurers, hospitals, and medical associations —at which the premiums and benefits for the next year are agreed.

## Patients' contributions

Patients make some direct contribution to the costs of their care in

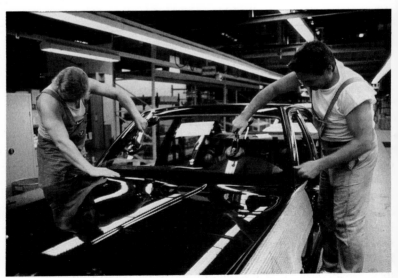

Car workers in Germany contribute 6% of earnings for health insurance; their employers pay in another 6% on their behalf

all countries in the OECD. In some this simply takes the form of a part payment for drugs. In several insurance schemes, however, such as in Belgium and France, the patient is required to pay a contribution—which may be as much as 25%—to the cost of a consultation with a general practitioner, and contributions are also required for hospital treatment. It is possible but not obligatory for citizens to insure against these direct payments. No direct charge is usually made to the elderly, the chronic sick, or the unemployed; and prolonged illness is never expensive in the way that it may be in the United States.

## Payments and fees

The ways in which doctors and hospitals are paid for the work they do also vary widely. Doctors working outside hospitals usually own the premises from which they practise or rent space in a health centre. Hospitals are owned and run almost exclusively by the state or by local government in most of the Scandinavian countries. Elsewhere in Europe some hospitals are state owned, some are run for profit by private companies, some are run by non-profit corporations, and some are owned and run by the insurance companies themselves. The proportion of hospitals owned and run by the state ranges from 50% in Germany, 66% in France, and 85% in Netherlands to virtually 100% in Sweden—though even in that temple of socialism there are a few private nursing homes.

The hospitals and the medical staff working in them may, as in Britain and Scandinavia, be financed from taxation, with the doctors earning salaries. In insurance based systems there is usually some link between payment and the work done, with the insurance funds paying either a daily rate or on an item of service basis. Some of the systems are of Byzantine complexity. In Germany, for example, under the statutory health insurance scheme "neither the patient nor the doctor knows at the time of treatment the exact amount that the doctor will be paid. The patient, moreover, will never know. The doctor will receive payment later through his professional association on the basis of an agreed nomenclature of services and in accordance with a scale of fees worked out on the basis of the forecast overall budget agreed by the funds and apportioned among the physicians within a region in relation to their workload."[1]

Doctors in general practice may be salaried, paid on a capitation basis, or paid per item of service or per patient treated—or they may be paid by a combination of these methods. In Netherlands, for example, the health insurance schemes fix an earnings target for general practitioners and calculate the capitation payment to provide 70% of this target. The assumption is that each doctor will earn the remaining 30% of the target from private practice, for which payment is made on an item of service basis.

## Actual health expenditure

The most widely used measures of health expenditure are the amount spent per person expressed in US dollars and the amount spent per person as a fraction of GDP (figure).[2] Neither measure gives a true picture of differences between countries in the health care delivered to the patient. Factors that also have to be taken into account include the expectations of and the demand by patients, how well doctors and other health workers are paid relative to the rest of the population, and the overall efficiency of the system—one recent estimate suggested that nearly a quarter of the expenditure on health care in the United States went on administrative costs.

What these measures do provide is some guidance on changes within and between countries. The past two decades have seen substantial growth in health expenditure in all countries with the

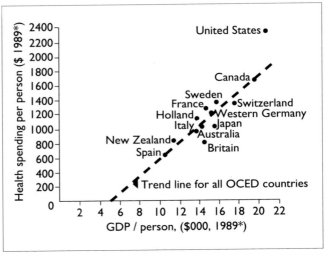

Health expenditure in OECD countries in US dollars and as proportion of gross domestic product

exception of those in Scandinavia, which has pulled back a little towards the average in the European Community. Health expenditure has grown in Britain, but the rate of growth has been slow compared with most of our neighbours; our overall expenditure is still near the bottom of the table.

1 Sandier S. Health services utilisation and physician income trends. *Health Care Financing Review* 1989;suppl:33-47.
2 Schieber GJ, Poullier J-P. International health spending: issues and trends. *Health Affairs* 1991 Spring:106-16.

# Medical education

STEPHEN BREARLEY

One of the principal objectives of the Treaty of Rome was the establishment of free migration within the European Economic Community (now the European Communities (EC)). Free migration implies a right to live and to work in any member state. For this to be practical for professional people a mechanism had to be found to recognise professional qualifications granted in one country in all the others. The first group for whom such a mechanism was set up was doctors, but it took 18 years from the signing of the treaty to agree the medical directives, which provide the essential framework.[1]

This delay was indicative of the diversity in medical training and qualifications which existed and still exists to a considerable extent in western Europe. Early negotiations on the directives sought to define precisely, in terms of duration and content, the training which doctors had to undergo if their qualifications were to be recognised throughout the community. An agreement of this nature proved impossible. It was the president of the European Commission, Ralf Dahrendorf, who cut the Gordian knot by declaring that, whatever their educational background, doctors throughout the community had similar skills and attributes and that, as the final product was the same, a qualification awarded by one member state should be regarded as satisfactory by all the others.

As a result the requirements of the directives, in terms of education leading to a basic medical qualification, are minimal (box). The directives have made free migration for doctors a reality but as a means of setting educational standards they have been a failure.

Mutual recognition of qualifications is a prerequisite for free migration because the titles attesting medical qualifications are legally protected in all EC states. Migrating doctors can practise only if their

30

The 1975 medical directives require that training leading to a recognised qualification should ensure:

- Adequate knowledge of the sciences on which medicine is based
- Sufficient understanding of the structure, functions, and behaviour of healthy and sick persons
- Adequate knowledge of clinical disciplines and practices
- Suitable clinical experience in hospitals under appropriate supervision.

Adequate, sufficient, suitable, and appropriate are not defined.

The 1975 medical directives require that training leading to a recognised specialist qualification must:

- Include practical and theoretical instruction
- Be a full time course, recognised by the competent authority*
- Be held in approved premises
- Involve personal participation by the trainee in the work of the establishment
- Last for a stipulated minimum duration.

*Provision for part time training was made in a 1982 directive.

qualifications are recognised as giving them a right to that title. In many states the title medical specialist is also legally protected. This is a consequence of the reimbursement arrangements of social security systems, which differ for specialists and generalists. In order to enable specialists to migrate it was necessary for the directives to include provisions for the mutual recognition of specialist qualifications.

These provisions are almost as weak as those governing basic medical qualifications (box). In those countries where protected specialist titles exist the period of postgraduate training leading to them is normally between three and six years. This is reflected in the directives. Although the minimal standards of training required are comfortably exceeded in almost all EC states, they are probably not achieved in a minority.

There is widespread misunderstanding of the meaning of mutual recognition of specialist qualifications. The directives require each country to recognise the named qualifications in specialised medicine awarded in other member states: countries must give these named qualifications the same effect as they give to their own qualifications. This effect, where it exists, has to do with reimbursement arrangements under social security systems. Such a system does not exist in

Principal recommendations of the Advisory Committee on Medical Training, 1978, 1982, and 1985:

• Each state should have a competent authority to determine standards, inspect and recognise training centres, coordinate basic with specialist training, award certificates attesting legal qualification, and establish relations with corresponding bodies in other member states
• Trainee numbers must be related to training facilities and to the future need for specialists
• Remunerated, full time training with a service element is the norm
• Trainees must progressively assume a greater degree of independent responsibility as their skill and experience grow
• Training should proceed via a common trunk from the general to the more specialised.

the United Kingdom, where the title of specialist is not legally protected. Consequently, there is no effect to be given to a specialist title carried by a doctor from elsewhere.

The United Kingdom specialist qualification listed in the directives is the certificate of specialist training which may be issued by the General Medical Council to appropriately trained British doctors who wish to work as specialists in other member states. Like all the other listed specialist qualifications it is without effect in the United Kingdom. Furthermore, fellowships and memberships of royal colleges, higher degrees, and certificates of accreditation are not among the qualifications listed in the directives and have no status elsewhere in the European Community.

## Basic medical training

Luxemburg has no medical school. All the remaining countries claim to have a numerus clausus, or numerical limit on medical school places, but determine it in different ways. In Italy there is practically no restriction on entry to the course and there have been examples of as many as 2000 in a class. France exercises control by means of an examination at the end of the first year, with only 20% of students being admitted to the remainder of the course, and there is a process of continuous attrition in Belgium. All other countries exercise control at entry. The number of places is rarely related to expected demand for doctors and bears a variable relation to the educational capacity of the schools.

Where selection at entry is practised, school leaving grades are always an important criterion but various other factors may be taken into account. In Germany candidates accumulate additional points for the time they have been waiting for a place and for their assessment at interview. Spain has a national examination (selectividad), the results of which are combined with school grades. In Netherlands there is a lottery which is weighted in favour of those with better school results.

In all countries the course lasts at least six years (the preregistration year in the United Kingdom is part of basic medical education), corresponding to the requirements of the directives (six years or 5500 hours of instruction). Generally, it is divided into preclinical and clinical components, but the proportions vary. The amount of laboratory work in the preclinical period varies and in countries with large medical school intakes it is virtually non-existent.

In many countries the clinical period is still largely theoretical and nowhere do students spend as much time in clinical areas as in the United Kingdom and the Republic of Ireland. Discussions with trainees from EC countries suggest that, typically, patient contact represents 20% of a student's time in Italy, three hours a day in Spain, four to six hours a week in Germany. In Belgium much clinical training is by means of patient demonstrations. In general, clinicians seem to show less interest in teaching students at the bedside than they do in the United Kingdom. Almost all countries confine teaching exclusively to university hospitals.

Most medical schools assess their students by in course examinations, frequently numerous. In some countries these are entirely theoretical (written or oral) and in most others testing of clinical skills plays only a small part.

Variability is at its greatest with regard to general clinical training (the preregistration year in the United Kingdom). A comparable period exists in the Republic of Ireland, Denmark, France, and, since 1988, in Germany. In other countries the last year of the medical course constitutes a form of internship but with much less responsibility than is borne by house officers in the United Kingdom. Greek doctors are required to complete one year of government service, usually in singlehanded practice providing care to rural communities, before being eligible to apply for specialist training.

## Specialist training

In all countries the nature of specialist training reflects the form of the health service. In the United Kingdom, where specialist practice is conducted almost exclusively by consultants in the NHS, training is designed to produce individuals with the skills, knowledge, and experience necessary for appointment as a consultant. Most other European countries have a social security system, under which most specialists are in private practice outside hospitals, are approached directly by patients, provide a largely outpatient service, and recoup their fees through the system. Such an arrangement demands a means whereby the public and the social security system can identify a qualified specialist but it does not require a training as prolonged and exhaustive as is usual in the United Kingdom because the responsibilities of specialists are different. Qualification as a specialist does not indicate suitability for appointment to a senior hospital and is perhaps better compared with acquiring the fellowship of the Royal College of Surgeons or the membership of the Royal College of Physicians. For those wishing to pursue a career in hospital medicine further training and experience are necessary.

Because specialist qualifications have a legal meaning within social security systems the training programme leading to them in many countries is also statutory. Authority thus rests with governments, though the system is normally operated by medical bodies. This is in marked contrast to the United Kingdom, where medical bodies have almost complete freedom to determine the duration and content of training.

Minimum training times in the community are set out in the table. In most countries, but not in the United Kingdom, a single programme provides the trainee with the complete training, which may involve rotation between departments but rarely between hospitals. The

Duration of specialist training in the European Community in a range of specialties*

| Specialty | Years | |
|---|---|---|
| | Minimum | Actual range |
| Anaesthetics | 3 | 3-6 |
| General surgery | 5 | 5-6 |
| Orthopaedics | 5 | 5-6 |
| Ophthalmology | 3 | 3-4 |
| Obstetrics and gynaecology | 4 | 4-6 |
| Internal medicine | 5 | 5-6 |
| Paediatrics | 4 | 4-5 |
| Psychiatry | 4 | 4-5·5 |

*Excludes United Kingdom and Republic of Ireland.

United Kingdom and France are the only countries in which the number of programmes is related to the anticipated need for specialists. Other countries are moving in this direction but, in general, there is a considerable overproduction of specialists.

Entry to training is by a competitive grading examination in France and Spain. Elsewhere, trainees have to apply for posts and there is considerable competition. There is good evidence in Germany that some trainees are working unpaid in the hope of obtaining a post when one becomes vacant, and in several countries trainees may have to wait for several years before being accepted.

Training is normally provided in paid posts involving clinical responsibility under supervision but this is still not the case in Italy, where specialist training is conceived as a taught course in a university. Because the number of trainees is often large, practical experience may be slight. In Greece the official ratio of one trainee for every three beds is not universally maintained. Most countries have a list of recognised trainers or institutions, often laying down criteria for such recognition, but regular inspection of training posts occurs only in the United Kingdom and Netherlands. Paid study leave is exceptional.

Satisfactory completion of the programme is normally attested by the trainer, though Belgium and Luxemburg also require trainees to present log books of their experience. There is an exit examination in Germany, Italy, and Greece.

## Training general practitioners

In the United Kingdom general practice is the only medical discipline in which completion of a specific training is a legal requirement. Similar requirements exist in Denmark, Netherlands, and France, while voluntary training schemes exist in several other countries. As the result of a 1986 directive such training will become mandatory throughout the community for doctors wishing to establish themselves in general medical practice after 31 December 1994.[2] The directive requires at least one year of training in hospital posts and one year in a recognised practice.

This directive represents a genuine advance in training standards but several countries are experiencing difficulties with its implementation. Because of the intense competition for training posts in hospitals it has not been possible to reserve a sufficient number for those intending a career in general practice, and not all governments have been prepared to fund the general practice component. The Union

Européen des Médecins Omnipraticiens, which represents general practitioners, believes that the training should, in any case, be of three years' duration. These problems remain to be overcome.

## Keeping up to date

Throughout Europe specialists have long been involved in continuing medical education by means of specialist societies and journals and through contact with colleagues and trainees. Until recently general practitioners have been much more isolated and lacked educational opportunities. The ethical duty of both groups to involve themselves in continuing education has been recognised by their representative organisations, though any form of compulsion has been stoutly rejected.

Provision for continuing medical education has improved in the past decade. Several countries have legislated for its establishment, and others have introduced voluntary machinery. Italy is the only country in which participation is mandatory and backed by financial sanctions, but no provision for the necessary courses has been made.

## Advisory Committee on Medical Training

The first two medical directives were accompanied by a third establishing the Advisory Committee on Medical Training within the European Commission "to help ensure a comparably demanding standard of training in (all member states of) the community."[3] This body, comprising nominated experts drawn from the competent authorities, the universities, and the profession in equal numbers, has published three reports on the problems of specialist training. Some of its recommendations are set out in the box.[4-6]

Sadly, these recommendations have not been widely implemented, and the European Commission has not been prepared to bring them forward in the form of new directives. A major obstacle to progress has been the lack of an educational infrastructure in several countries, where even the requirements of the existing directives may not be fulfilled in their entirety. Where training is largely a government rather than a professional responsibility, as in Greece, or wholly in the hands of the universities, as in Italy, doctors have not been able to bring about changes which many see as desirable.

In 1987 the Permanent Working Group of European Junior Hospital Doctors found that the advisory committee's recommendations were

Principal recommendations of the Permanent Working Group of European Junior Hospital Doctors, adopted 1988:

- The recommendations of the Advisory Committee on Medical Training should be supported and implemented
- Each trainee should at all times have a clearly identified trainer with defined responsibilities
- Training should include practical and theoretical instruction, private study and research, regular critical scrutiny with unambiguous feedback, and career guidance
- Trainers should receive training in educational methods and guidance on the fulfilment of their task
- Training posts should be inspected by the training authorities at least every five years
- The quality of training, rather than an exit examination, should be the means to achieving high standards, since examinations cannot test the full range of skills and attributes required in a specialist.

not fulfilled in their entirety in any member state.[7] Particularly common were the absence of any system for inspection of training posts, lack of regulation of trainee numbers, scarcity of part time training, and inadequate supervision of trainees. The permanent working group adopted a policy statement on postgraduate medical education in 1988, the first such document to have been written by trainees, addressing educational issues which had not been dealt with by the advisory committee (box).[7] Although well received and forwarded to the commission by the Standing Committee of Doctors of the EC, this document seems destined to have even less effect than its predecessors.

## Future prospects

Standards of medical training, at both basic and specialist levels, remain variable across the community. Some of this variability is inevitable and perhaps desirable, given the different historical, social, and cultural influences which shape training systems, but some is due to political inertia, weak government, and lack of investment. Poor standards of training, combined with the overproduction of doctors, undermine the principle of a free market as well as threatening standards of patient care.

There is thus a case for reviewing the medical directives and strengthening their educational provisions. Such a move would require a lead from the commission, which has repeatedly stated that it does not seek to intervene in the funding or administration of national health care systems. Commissioner Papandreou recently indicated that the commission was seeking a greater role in the areas of prevention, care, and medical assistance and was setting up an informal health committee. Whether this might lead eventually to the setting up of a directorate for health and greater interest on the part of the commission in medical training remains to be seen but, in the short term, new measures do not seem likely.

Improvements in training are more likely to result from national initiatives and from the collaborative efforts of European medical bodies. Perhaps the most promising of these is the recent decision of the Union Européen des Médecins Specialistes, through its mono-specialty sections, to establish European boards, with the aim of harmonising specialist training. The boards will set training standards, inspect and recognise training programmes, and award certificates to those who complete training in a recognised centre. Because they will be part of the existing representative framework these boards are likely to be more credible and more effective than freestanding European colleges, which have also been proposed.

The other major influence for good is free migration. The number of doctors taking advantage of this is small, though substantial numbers are now coming to the United Kingdom, but Europe offers an unrivalled range of medical experience and an opportunity for the crossfertilisation of ideas. Sadly, migration for educational purposes has been hampered by the demand for posts generated by unemployment while exchange schemes have proved difficult to set up because of unequal standards of training, language barriers, and administrative complexity.

It is inevitable that training standards in Europe will converge, but they start from a point of great diversity and progress is likely to be slow. The United Kingdom has the advantage of a strong tradition of clinical teaching, a well established infrastructure, and an autonomous medical profession. It has much to offer to its partners in the community.

1 Council directives of 16 June 1975. 75/362/EEC and 75/363/EEC. *Official Journal of the European Communities* 1975;**L167**:1-16.
2 Council directive of 15 September 1986 on specific training in general medical practice. 86/457/ EEC. *Official Journal of the European Communities* 1986;**L267**:26-8.
3 Council directive of 15 June 1975 setting up an advisory committee on medical training. 75/364/ EEC. *Official Journal of the European Communities* 1975;**L167**:17-8.

4 Advisory Committee on Medical Training. *Report and recommendations on the general problems of specialist training.* Brussels: Commission of the European Communities, 1978.
5 Advisory Committee on Medical Training. *Second report and recommendations on the training of specialists.* Brussels: Commission of the European Communities, 1983.
6 Advisory Committee on Medical Training. *Third report and recommendations of the conditions for specialist training.* Brussels: Commission of the European Communities, 1986.
7 Brearley S, Beuzart S, Gredal J, Suntinger A, Gentleman D. Permanent Working Group of European Junior Hospital Doctors. Policy statement on postgraduate medical education. *Med Educ* 1989;**23**:339-47.

# Medical manpower

STEPHEN BREARLEY

Planning of medical manpower has been practised for decades in the United Kingdom. But this is not the case in many of its partners in the European Community (EC). Control of medical student numbers in line with the expected demand for doctors occurs in, at most, two other EC states (box) but in most of the rest there has been a substantial overproduction of doctors, which has led to considerable, and in some cases catastrophic, medical unemployment.

This is a matter of concern to British doctors for two reasons. Firstly, as a member of the European Community, the United Kingdom has implemented its medical directives, which give all doctors who are nationals of commuity countries and hold medical qualifications granted in those countries the right to practise anywhere in the community. Over 1000 such doctors are now coming to the United Kingdom each year, something that was not forseen when medical manpower was last scrutinised. Secondly, as a partner in the medical community of Europe, the United Kingdom has an interest in standards of training and practice throughout the EC and these are inevitably jeopardised where student and trainee numbers are excessive and many doctors have insufficient work.

To a greater or lesser degree these concerns are shared by all the medical associations in the EC. They were set out by the EC's standing committee of doctors in its 1985 Cannes declaration, which called for urgent measures to establish manpower planning machinery in all member states. In practice, the liberal constitutions adopted by several states after the second world war make the introduction of such measures difficult as they would infringe the guaranteed right of citizens to higher education. In general, medical manpower planning does not figure highly among the priorities of national governments or

40

**Determination of medical student numbers**

| | |
|---|---|
| Numerus clausus* related to manpower needs | Denmark |
| | United Kingdom |
| | (Finland) |
| | (Iceland) |
| | (Norway) |
| | (Sweden) |
| Numerus clausus* related to educational capacity of medical schools | Germany |
| | Ireland |
| | Netherlands |
| | Spain |
| | (Austria) |
| | (Switzerland) |
| Other control mechanism | Belgium |
| | France |
| No effective control | Greece |
| | Italy |
| No medical school | Luxemburg |

*Limitation of the number of medical school places.

the European Commission, and in the past 10 years only one country, France, has made a serious attempt to reduce its overproduction of doctors.

This ambivalence on the part of governments reflects the nature of most of the health care systems in Europe. Whereas the British government is a virtual monopoly employer of doctors and controls the number of posts available, most European doctors are in free practice, recouping their fees through a social security system. Any appropriately qualified doctor can set up a practice and so there is no fixed number of medical jobs. In such a system the demand for doctors cannot be measured and the supply tends to be left to market forces. This laissez faire approach has led to a trebling in the number of doctors in the 12 EC countries since the early 1950s.

## Inexact data

Where medical manpower planning is not practised reliable manpower data tend not to be collected. All data on manpower are therefore inexact, and such data as are available need to be interpreted with caution. National registers of doctors, such as that maintained by the General Medical Council, may not include retired doctors, unemployed doctors, or those who are not working for a variety of other reasons. Government data may relate only to doctors working in government funded posts or registered with the social security system. Even the definition of a doctor is variable. French internes are still technically students until they obtain their MD by thesis, usually three or four years after beginning their postgraduate training.

Several bodies have investigated EC medical manpower: the Statistical Office of the European Communities (1984), the Standing Committee of Doctors of the EC (1988), and the Permanent Working Group of European Junior Hospital Doctors (1991). The permanent working group's study, reported at a Symposium in Florence in October 1991 but so far unpublished, is the most comprehensive to date. A synopsis is given in table I.

No one knows how many doctors there are in Italy and Greece. No distinction was made between doctors and dentists in Italy until recently. There is practically no limit on the numbers admitted to medical school and, of those who obtain medical degrees, a considerable number never find medical work. Greece has a numerus clausus (a limit on the number of medical school places) but many of the

TABLE I — Medical demography of the European Community

| Country | Medical workforce | No of doctors per head of population | No (%) of unemployed doctors |
|---|---|---|---|
| Belgium | 35 000 | 290 | |
| Denmark | 14 505 | 340 | 70 (0·5) |
| France | 164 022 | 336 | 1 000 (0·6) |
| Germany | 192 480 | 332 | 15 400 (8·0) |
| Greece | 35 000 | 290 | 0 |
| Republic of Ireland | 5 571 | 628 | |
| Italy | 230 265 | 248 | 40 000 (17·3) |
| Luxemburg | 700 | 534 | |
| Netherlands | 29 867 | 492 | 600 (2·0) |
| Portugal | 24 503 | 389 | 0 |
| Spain | 131 684 | 296 | 6 000 (4·6) |
| United Kingdom | 101 396 | 562 | 300 (0·3) |
| Austria | 211 572 | 352 | 2 500 (9·0) |
| Finland | 12 317 | 402 | 0 |
| Iceland | 743 | 340 | 0 |
| Norway | 11 588 | 364 | 0 |
| Sweden | 23 565 | 360 | 0 |
| Switzerland | 20 584 | 321 | 620 (0·3) |

Greeks who obtain a medical degree bypass it by going abroad to begin their studies, usually in eastern Europe or Italy. They are then entitled to return to Greece to complete the course.

Germany is one of the countries that has difficulty in reducing its intake into medical schools for legal reasons. The number of places is fixed, but in relation to the educational capacity of the schools rather than to manpower needs. Because of Germany's size its overproduction in absolute numbers is among the largest in the community. Unemployment is growing rapidly, and some junior doctors are working without pay in the hope of furthering their training and ultimately obtaining a post. The largest group of continental doctors coming to the United Kingdom is German and, after reunification, the right to free migration is being extended to doctors from the former East Germany.

Free migration is also becoming available to doctors from Scandinavia, Austria, Switzerland, and Lichtenstein (the countries of the European Free Trade Association (EFTA)) as the result of the agreement creating a European economic space, which was signed in October. There are approximately one million doctors working in the EC and a further 100 000 in EFTA countries. The number of doctors in any country is, however, a meaningless figure unless related to population size. The number of inhabitants per doctor in each country is given in table I. This shows that medical density within the community varies almost threefold, with the highest densities occurring in countries with little control over medical student numbers and a high proportion of doctors in free practice. Not surprisingly, these are also the countries with the highest levels of medical unemployment and underemployment.

## Unemployment and underemployment

One of the problems that has bedevilled the study of medical manpower in Europe is the lack of agreed definitions of the terms used. In an attempt to overcome this the permanent working group has adopted the definitions of employment status set out in the box.

Underemployment is an unfamiliar term in the United Kingdom, but it is applicable to doctors without regular appointments who earn a living from a succession of locum posts, with intervening periods of unemployment. In Europe as a whole it more often applies to doctors in free practice who are consulted by few patients and may lose their skills as a result. They may supplement their incomes by doing non-

**Employment status**

*Unemployment:* A doctor is unemployed when, on a specified date, he or she is eligible to practise but is involuntarily without any form of remunerative work.

*Misemployment:* A doctor is misemployed when, on a specific date, he or she is eligible to practise, is unable to find work as a doctor, but obtains an income by working in a capacity not requiring a medical qualification.

*Underemployment:* A doctor is underemployed if he or she is unable to find medical work during part of the normal working week or if he or she is unable to find sufficient medical work to yield a remuneration appropriate to his or her experience and seniority.

*Long term unemployment* A doctor is long term unemployed when, while having been eligible to practise, he or she has been involuntarily without any remunerative medical work for a continuous period exceeding six calendar months.

Source: Permanent Working Group of European Junior Hospital Doctors (1988).

medical work. Because established posts are the exception in many countries, underemployment is often a bigger problem than unemployment.

Both unemployment and underemployment are extremely difficult to quantify, even in countries with good data on medical manpower. The number of unemployed and underemployed doctors in the United Kingdom is unknown, though it is believed to be low. The best available estimates for EC and EFTA countries are set out in table I, but it is unlikely that reliable figures can ever be obtained. Furthermore, it is questionable whether the holder of a medical qualification who has never practised and who earns a living outside medicine should still be counted as a doctor. It is possible, however, using computer modelling techniques, to make projections for the supply of and demand for doctors and to derive trends in unemployment. This approach has been adopted in the permanent working group's study and the result is surprising. The present high level of medical unemployment is attributable to a large and uncontrolled increase in medical school output in the 1960s and '70s. The corollary of this is that there will be a boom in medical retirements after the turn of the century. The size of the medical workforce may decrease and there may be a shortage of doctors.

These findings are reassuring in that the upward trend in unemployment seems to be part of a cyclical rather than an inexorable process. Equally, the possibility of a shortage of doctors should give pause for thought to health service planners, particularly in Britain, where there is not a surplus at present. Unfortunately, improvement is likely to come too late to help those doctors, now in their 30s and 40s, who make up the bulk of the unemployed and underemployed and who are likely to remain a lost generation.

## Hours of work

Despite the existence of serious medical unemployment, doctors throughout Europe continue to work substantially longer hours than other groups of workers. Once again, study of this question is hampered by the absence of agreed definitions. Hours of work are an issue chiefly for salaried doctors, who are predominantly trainees, but the method by which their hours are counted and remunerated differs from country to country.

A survey of junior doctors' hours of work was carried out under the auspices of the permanent working group in 1987 and data have also been collected by the Standing Committee of Doctors of the EC. The results show, not unexpectedly, that trainees in the United Kingdom have the longest hours of work in western Europe (table II). The shortest hours are found in Scandinavia, where several countries have a legal limit on the hours that may be worked. Even where hours are substantially shorter than in the United Kingdom they are often considered to be too long. Junior doctors in Netherlands have been engaged in acrimonious negotiations with their government on this subject.

Shorter hours are made possible in other countries by three factors. There are more doctors per head of population, trainee numbers are not restricted in line with expected demand for specialists, and the trainees tend to be concentrated in university hospitals or comparable institutions. Specialists in non-training hospitals enjoy little or no junior support but these hospitals do much less emergency work. It is interesting to speculate whether the United Kingdom will have to emulate its neighbours in any of these respects if the intractable problem of hours of work is to be solved.

TABLE II — Weekly hours of duty of junior doctors

| Hours of duty | Country |
|---|---|
| 40-49 | Italy<br>Luxemburg |
| 50-59 | Belgium<br>Denmark<br>Finland<br>Iceland<br>Norway<br>Sweden<br>Switzerland |
| 60-69 | Netherlands<br>Portugal<br>Spain |
| 70-79 | Ireland<br>Iceland |
| More than 80 | United Kingdom |

Sources: Survey of junior doctors' hours by Permanent Working Group of European Junior Hospital Doctors (1987), Standing Committee of Doctors of the EC's questionnaire on medical demography (1988).

## Older doctors and more women

The proportion of doctors who are women has increased steadily in all European countries. Women currently comprise 28% of the EC medical workforce but a half of those graduating from medical schools. By 2000 approximately one third of practising doctors will be women.

The age structure of the medical profession is much less uniform. Many countries experienced a boom in medical school output in the 1960s and '70s, followed by a gradual decline in the '80s, and where this occurred there is a progressive right shift of the age distribution curve with time.

The proportion of specialists in each country was included in the EC Statistical Office's 1984 report. Fewer than 30% of doctors are specialists in the United Kingdom, the Republic of Ireland, and Denmark, compared with 45-70% in other EC countries, but these figures should be interpreted with caution. In countries where free practice is predominant many specialists practise from their own offices, do not have admitting rights to hospitals, do not carry out invasive treatments, and often provide a degree of general medical service. Patients refer themselves directly to the doctor of their choice, specialist or generalist, and there is intense competition between the two groups for the same patients.

## Prospects for medical migration

The United Kingdom has seen a large increase in medical immigration from other EC countries in recent years, but it would be wrong to suppose that similar movements are being seen elsewhere. The United Kingdom is uniquely attractive to medical migrants because employment prospects, at least at senior house officer level, are better than anywhere else and because most doctors know English, the international language of medicine. Entry to specialist training is relatively easy, competition becoming more intense with increasing seniority, whereas in most other European countries there is fierce competition for entry to training programmes but progress thereafter is much more assured.

The 1989 medical manpower census for England and Wales identified 418 junior doctors born in the Republic of Ireland and 935 born in other EC countries. A survey carried out by the Department of Health in 1990 obtained responses from 622 non-Irish EC doctors. Over three quarters were from western Germany (42%), Netherlands (22%), or Spain (15%). Almost all (89%) were working as house officers or senior house officers. Eighteen per cent intended to settle permanently in the United Kingdom and a further 8% were undecided. Past experience suggests that the number who settle may prove to be greater than the number who came with that intention. It is not yet clear how successful those who attempt to return home will be in finding the posts they are seeking.

The number of British doctors who migrate to other European states is small (perhaps 50 a year, mostly for short periods) and no other country has reported medical migration on a large scale. The numbers migrating are, in fact, disappointingly small. The EC offers an unparalleled range of medical experience, and several bodies have tried to promote short term migration for educational purposes. These initiatives have largely been frustrated by the pressure on posts created by widespread unemployment.

The position is likely to change appreciably in the forseeable future. In the short term the permanent working group's study suggests that unemployment will get worse in those countries where it is already severe, but the United Kingdom may be short of several thousand doctors by the year 2000. This shortfall is likely to be made up by immigration from countries with high unemployment. In the next century, as medical manpower passes from surplus to deficit, immigration is likely to decline and opportunities abroad may increase. There may be an acute shortage of doctors in the United Kingdom unless corrective action is taken in good time.

# Who speaks for whom?

TESSA RICHARDS

British doctors are waking up to Europe with a vengeance. Interest has been fuelled by many factors: the broadening and deepening of the European Community; the single market[1]; the oversupply of doctors and wide discrepancies in standards of training[2]; trends in medical migration[3]; and patients crossing borders for treatment. The list goes on, but for whatever reasons all sections of the medical profession have set up European committees and are setting about influencing Brussels.

Those very few doctors who have been concerned with European medical affairs for decades have been cynically shaking their heads about this new found enthusiasm, but arguably it is a healthy sign. With the myriad of challenges and opportunities that the changing shape of Europe will bring there has never been a more important time for doctors to be aware of what is going on in the European Community.

The long established European medical bodies have been working for years, but new converts to Europe are concerned that they lack influence. The number of draft directives affecting health that have emerged after little discussion with doctors supports this view. The profession's voice has barely been heard among the cacophony of lobby groups in Brussels. Why this should be is unclear. Some are convinced that it is because the profession has lacked a substantive base in Brussels. Others cite personal and organisational factors. This article addresses these questions by taking a critical look at the bodies that represent or are seeking to represent doctors in Europe.

49

# Standing Committee of Doctors of the EC— An organisation at war with itself?

Established in 1959 the standing committee or comité permanent (CP), which is an independent voluntary organisation, is the only body that claims to represent all doctors in all member states of the EC. It is the last common path to the European Commission for statements which it and other medical groups, who send liaison officers to its meetings, formulate. This puts it in a unique position of power and responsibility (figure).

Membership is large—each of the 12 member states send several delegates from their representative medical organisations. Numbers are swelled by observers from Austria, Switzerland, Finland, Cyprus, and Hungary. The British contingent is represented by the British Medical Association and consists of (by accident rather than by design) an occupational physician, a gynaecologist, a general practitioner, a public health physician, and a junior doctor, supported by members of the BMA's European division.

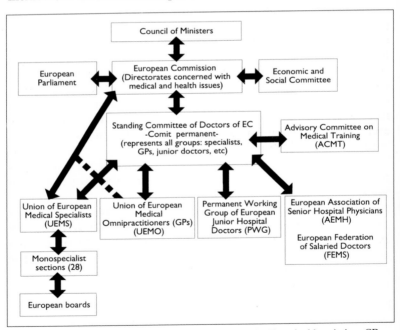

The Standing Committee of Doctors of EC—known by its French abbreviation, CP— has a unique position of power and responsibility

Costs are borne by the various medical associations, with each member state paying a weighted proportion. The BMA's share is 17%, which in 1991 amounted to about £60 000; simultaneous translations at meetings, mountains of paperwork, maintaining a secretariat, travel and accommodation expenses, and generous entertainment do not come cheap.

The standing committee's aims are to represent the medical profession of all member states; study and promote high standards of medical practice and health care; and promote free movement of doctors. As evidence of its success in meeting these objectives it can cite its role in shaping the original doctors' directives on mutual recognition of diplomas and the directives on vocational training in general practice. It can also point to numerous impressive sounding charters, statements, and recommendations that it has sent to the commission on subjects ranging from patients' right to choose their own doctor to the ethical obligations of professionals to keep up to date.

But making sound statements is not enough. Who listens? Many members of the standing committee admit, both in private and on paper, that the organisation lacks any stature in Brussels and has been ineffective in getting its views across to the decision makers.[4] Part of the problem is structural; the three year rotating presidency has ensured discontinuity since the secretariat is always changing from country to country, and the organisation has never had a fixed abode. Overlong agendas, indifferent chairmanship, few visible in house rules of debate, and unconcealed hostility and unproductive exchanges between national delegations have at times meant that meetings achieve little.

In recognition of these problems the standing committee—in response to an initiative generated by a British, French, and German working party—has opened a permanent office in Brussels and is in the process of revising its working practices.[5] Whether these moves (which will add to the costs) will make a difference is not clear. Views circulating at the committee's last meeting such as "It's all too little too late" and "Nothing much will be achieved if the right calibre of people are not there" seem to be widely held.

## European union of medical specialists—taking Euro qualifications too far?

The European Union of Medical Specialists (UEMS) can claim the

51

distinction of being the oldest body representing doctors in Europe. Unlike the standing committee it has a permanent secretariat in Brussels. In addition to its central management council it has 28 different monospecialist sections. New sections can be set up only if the specialty concerned is recognised in at least eight member states, and some sections function a good deal more efficiently than others. Associate membership of UEMS is held by some non-EC countries, including Austria, Finland, and Switzerland. The organisation is funded by contributions from member associations, which in Britain's case include the BMA, royal colleges, and specialist associations.

The aim of UEMS is to study issues related to specialist training and practice. In response to an edict from the commission to, in effect get its act together to do something about the variable standards of specialist training in Europe, it has agreed on an ambitious harmonisation programme. Its chosen approach is to get the monospecialist committees to set up European "boards" whose objective is to establish common criteria in the EC for training. Setting exit exams is deemed by some to be an inherent part of ensuring common standards, and the plastic surgeons and urologists, for example, are already in a position to hold their first exams. How necessary it is or might become for candidates to sit these expensive "voluntary" Euro exams is not clear.

In common with the standing committee, UEMS has serious organisational problems, the chief one being the gulf between its central management committee and the monospecialist sections. The membership of the central committee is not considered to be sufficiently representative of the organisation as a whole—(Britain is currently represented by the gynaecologist who is on the standing committee, a general surgeon, and a neurosurgeon). Repeatedly the specialist groups agree on a common line of action, only to find their views ignored or "misrepresented" at the centre. At the central committee's last meeting in Athens in September, for example, a motion that only doctors should be able to prescribe glasses got accepted. This is scarcely the accepted view among ophthalmologists, but with none present the dissenters could not generate enough momentum to throw the motion out.

Frustrations such as these have led some specialist groups to strike off on their own. Thus the anaesthetists have set up their own European body, which is already running regular specialist exams,[6] and the orthopaedic surgeons look set to follow suit.

## European union of general practitioners — pushing vocational training hard

The European Union of General Practitioners (UEMO) was set up in 1967 to raise standards of practice, training, and patient care. It is also concerned to "defend the role" of general practitioners as well as further their ethical, scientific, professional, social, and economic interests. British representation is shared between the BMA (General Medical Services Committee) and the Royal College of General Practitioners. The presidency and secretariat rotate between member state organisations on a four year basis.

UEMO's current concerns include the use of computers in general practice, quality assurance, training "trainers," and producing publications (box). It also has good links with some of the European Commission's research programmes including Europe Against Cancer and Advanced Informatics in Medicine. In conjunction with others it established the 1986 vocational training directive, which stipulates a minimum training period of two years for all general practitioners in the EC. It is now campaigning for an extension to three years, but this will be an uphill struggle. Some EC member states, notably Germany, have not yet got their two year vocational training schemes established.

## Permanent working group of junior hospital doctors — few grey hairs, more enthusiasm

The Permanent Working Group of European Junior Hospital Doctors (PWG) was set up in 1976 to improve relations among junior doctors in Europe and to exchange information on topics of mutual interest such as medical education, specialist training, and working conditions. Its membership is not confined to EC countries. Austria, Finland, Iceland, Norway, Sweden, and Switzerland are also represented, and observers from eastern Europe have attended recent meetings. In common with the other specialist European organisations described above, the BMA nominates representatives and bears a share of the costs (which are much less than those of the standing committee). EC member states host these meetings on a rotational basis.

An active organisation, PWG has produced several useful publications (box) and in common with UEMS and UEMO channels its policy statements to the commission largely through the standing

---

**Some publications on the European Community**

British Medical Association. *European communities. General guidance for doctors.* London: BMA, 1990.

British Medical Association. *European Community medical bodies. General information for doctors.* London: BMA, 1991.

British Medical Association. *Health care systems and professional organisations in the European Community.* London: BMA, 1991.

Permanent Working Group of European Junior Hospital Doctors. *Guide to health in Europe.* Paris: Impact Médecin, 1992.

Owen R, Dynes M. *The Times guide to 1992. Britain in a Europe without frontiers.* London: Times Books, 1989.

*Vachers' European companion and consultants' register.* Berkhamsted: Vachers, 1991.

Ramsay A. *European communities information.* London: AAL Publishing, 1990.

Budd S, Jones A. *The EEC: a guide to the maze.* 3rd ed. London: Kogan Page, 1989.

Office for Official Publications of the European Communities. *The European Community as a publisher.* London: HMSO, 1990.

European Union of General Practitioners. *The position of the general medical practitioner and general practice in the health care systems of the European Community.* London: BMA, 1986.

*EuroBrief.* Monthly digest of European medical affairs available from the BMA's Professional, Scientific, and International Affairs Division.

*A guide to the registration requirements for doctors of the European communities and information concerning access to medical practice in the social security systems. 1985.* (Excludes Spain, Portugal, and Greece.) Available from the BMA's Professional, Scientific, and International Affairs Division.

---

committee. At the latter's meeting in Madrid in September the PWG expressed its suspicion about the proposed exit exams on the grounds that passing them would not guarantee competence and they might at some stage be used to exclude or limit the numbers of aspiring specialists. The group's main concern of late, however, has been medical manpower in Europe, and its findings were aired at the group's symposium in Florence last October.[7]

## Advisory committee on medical training — starved of resources

The Advisory Committee on Medical Training was created in 1975

---

**Where to go for further information**

*Official Journal of the European Communities* is published monthly and is available from HMSO.

BMA European Communities Committee
BMA House
Tavistock Square
London WC1H 9JP
(tel 071 387 4499)

The secretariat will answer queries from members about medicine and the EC.

Commission of the European Communities
8 Storey's Gate
London SW1P 3AT
(tel 071 222 8122)

The press office provides information on all aspects of the EC.

United Kingdom Office of the European Parliament
2 Queen Anne's Gate
London SW1
(tel 071 222 0411)

---

by the European Commission. Based in Brussels and funded by the commission (via Directorate General III), this statutory organisation has a much closer relation with commission staff than any of the other European medical groups, and its views are taken seriously. Nominations to the committee, which is made up of three members from each member state, are made by national governments on the advice of "appropriate" bodies. In Britain's case this once again includes the BMA.

Originally concerned with standards of undergraduate training, the committee has now turned its attention to postgraduate training as well and spurred the current wave of activity related to the European boards. Given its standing, the advisory committee ought to be in a strong position to push through improved standards of medical training. Unfortunately it is not. Gross underfunding coupled with the constantly changing membership have left it struggling to fulfil its role.

## Other European groups representing doctors

Other specialised medical groups representing doctors' interests in

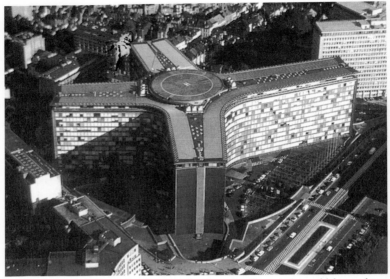

The Berlaymont in Brussels—home to the European Commission, which now has a formal mandate to draft legislation on health[7] is increasing steadily

Europe include the Conférence Internationale des Ordres, the European Federation of Salaried Doctors, and the European Association of Senior Hospital Physicians. Each sends a representative to the standing committee's meetings. Details of their structure and objectives are set out in a booklet available from the BMA.[8]

## The British and Europe

Apart from being the key source of nominations to the main European organisations that represent doctors (CP, UEMS, UEMO, PWG), the BMA "monitors European affairs" via its European Communities Committee and advises Council on the implications of EC proposals for draft legislation. It also produces publications and *Euro Brief*, a monthly bulletin on European affairs. By virtue of its membership of the European organisations described above it keeps a close finger on the pulse of their activities. Over the years it has exerted influence on many issues, including the free movement of doctors and vocational training in Europe. The BMA's parliamentary unit is also seeking to strengthen its contacts with Brussels, especially with members of the European Parliament so that it can increase its currently very limited lobbying powers in Europe. Approval and financial backing have been gained for a European office, and the organisation now employs a professional consultant based in Brussels.

## The royal colleges

At the conference of medical royal colleges and their faculties last April the decision was made to set up another European committee. The justification for this, according to the new committee's chairman, is that doctors' representation in Europe, as stage managed by the BMA, has been too narrow.

The aims of the Conference of Medical Royal Colleges European Committee (CRCECt) include the need to define what constitutes a specialist. Not as easy as it sounds, given that some countries, such as Britain, have no set definitions while the Italians boast over 130 different specialties. The committee is also keen to promote more movement of hospital doctors within Europe, especially at registrar level. As a prelude to this it encourages language training for doctors. It also sees itself (ambitiously if not arrogantly) as a role model "for the future development of medical services and postgraduate training and to promote the professional and scientific image embodied by the royal colleges. Also to advise on the creation of parallel institutions in other EC countries as required."

The Royal College of General Practitioners, through its international committee, has been monitoring EC developments for a good deal longer, and has good relations with existing European organisations including the Leeuwenhorst Group (a European think tank for general practice), the World Association of Colleges and Academies of General Practice, WHO Europe, and the International Society of General Practice. Recently it has been concerned with projects to help develop primary care in Romania and Czechoslovakia.

Not to be outdone, the Royal College of Surgeons and the Royal College of Physicians have also set up European committees but their prime role is organising "European" scientific meetings and exchange visits. The Royal Society of Medicine's European Group has a similar role.

## Conclusion

If the number of committees representing doctors in Europe bore a direct relation to the effectiveness of that representation, British doctors and their European colleagues could rest easy in their beds. Sadly this is not the case. Some of the organisations have serious internal problems and the communication between them is not ideal. Inevitably there has been duplicated effort and some rivalry, but the key problem has been that none of the individual groups has achieved sufficient credibility in Brussels. This has meant that the European Commission, which is swamped with information from what it regards as "unrecognised sources," has lent little credence to their views, however sound and however passionately couched. Furthermore, at times the groups have great difficulty actually reaching a common view. This is unsurprising and not unique to medicine; political and cultural divides are large, and no doubt agreement will become increasingly difficult as the EC enlarges.

Although it may not be easy to influence the Brussels bureaucracy, it is not impossible. Organisations such as Greenpeace and Friends of the Earth, who campaign on environmental issues, seem to have got lobbying down to a fine art. Similarly, the European Citizen Action Bureau, which has been running for only a few years, has made an impact and is a fund of useful information on many issues including health.[9] Being based in Brussels obviously helps, and in many ways it is extraordinary that it has taken the medical profession so long to recognise this. Having enough people of the right calibre is also important. That the British view has for so long been entrusted to so few may have had the merit of ensuring some continuity but it also suggests a lack of vision, stemming in part from the profession's relative indifference to Europe.

New European enthusiasts are surely welcome, but they will do the profession little favour if they do not coordinate their activities and work with rather than against the established European bodies. All need to keep sight of the need to campaign for improved standards of health care in the community as a whole, as well as for the self interest of the profession.

1 Leidl R. How will the single European market affect health care? *BMJ* 1991;**303**:1081-2.
2 Brearley S, Gentleman D. Doctors and the European Community. *BMJ* 1991;**302**:1221-2.
3 Richards T. Euromigration. *BMJ* 1991;**302**:1296-7.
4 Beecham L. BMA to help reform doctors' EC committee. *BMJ* 1990;**301**:935.
5 Richards T. Brussels base for EC doctors. *BMJ* 1991;**303**:877.
6 Editorial. European diploma in anaesthetics and intensive care. *Lancet* 1991; **338**:219.
7 Beecham L. Ray of hope on European manpower. *BMJ* 1991;**303**:1220.
8 Euro-citizen-action-service. The European Citizen; Health. *European Citizens Week* 1991:No 10. (16-20 September.)

# Nursing in Europe

KIRSTEN STALLKNECHT

When discussion began among European professional groups about harmonising educational standards the anxiety was that member states would be asked to change their individual systems to a standardised European version. Attitudes changed, however, as a result of the Dahrendorf hearing in 1973, when the ministers of education decided that instead of a general harmonising of education the new approach should be the establishment of a set of minimum standards. This would simplify and speed up the process of allowing the free movement of people and services within the European community (EC).

This new approach forced the professional associations representing nurses and other health professionals to reassess their attitudes, but these organisations were still mostly concerned with protecting their own interests rather than with the advancement of the unity of the EC. Mostly, too, they continued to believe that the system in their own country was the best.

The EC agreed directives for many professions in the 1970s, and

---

**Nursing numbers**

No reliable statistics on nurses and nursing personnel are available for the EC, but some figures can be extracted from the Vienna conference material. The general trend in Europe is for continuing growth in the demand for nurses, but demographic changes will make satisfaction of this demand difficult. The European office of WHO has estimated that 21 European countries will have less than 30% of their population under 20 years by the year 2000. Only six countries are expected to see a rise in the numbers of young people. At the same time the numbers of old people will continue to grow.

---

doctors and nurses were among these. Nevertheless it was the political decision to form a single market that gave real, practical importance to the concept of free movement. We now need to recognise that the Europe of the 1990s is changing dramatically—and that developments in the Eastern bloc states will force even further changes. In the long run the living and working conditions, the health and education services, and so on cannot be allowed to differ as widely as at present between eastern and western Europe.

## Nurses' cooperation

In the late 1960s the nurses of Europe began to meet and eventually formed a group of nurses' associations in the EC member countries and countries applying for membership. The Standing Committee of Nurses of the EC (PCN) was formally established in 1971. Its main task was to promote better educational standards for nurses in the EC and—especially after the Dahrendorf hearing—to help develop directives on general nursing education and the free movement of nurses in Europe. Considerable differences were soon apparent in the educational systems, and the first task of the PCN was to agree a set of common minimum requirements to be implemented through the directives. These requirements were met in 1977 with two directives, 452 and 453, on "the mutual recognition of diplomas, certificates and other evidence of the formal qualifications of nurses responsible for general care" and "the coordination of provisions laid down by law, regulation, or administrative action in respect of the activities of nurses responsible for general care."

In some countries this agreement on minimum standards led to improvements in the standard of education for nurses; in others it left education unchanged. The main fear among the leaders of European nurses had been that the minimum standards would prevent the more advanced countries from developing better educational programmes. In practice this has not proved to be so. In most of the countries of the EC educational programmes have continued to evolve and improve.

## General development

Once the PCN had been formed it seemed natural for nurses to extend their cooperation to other areas. One problem with this project was that general statistics on nursing and nurses proved not to be available. Indeed they are still not available in a form suitable for the

PCN to embark on planning for the future. Nevertheless, some progress has been made. One valuable initiative has been the work done by the European office of the World Health Organisation on nursing as part of the health field. The WHO's medium term programme in nursing and midwifery has inspired the leaders of European nurses, and the "Health for All" programme has encouraged nurses to take a much more active role in health planning and promotion. This was very apparent at the WHO European nursing conference in Vienna in 1988, when a joint declaration on nursing and nursing education in Europe was adopted unanimously by the representatives from all European countries.[1] The role of the nurse was defined at the meeting as one based on a generalist training with strong links with primary health care and with the possibility of further education in various clinical specialty fields, in management, education, and research.

The minimum requirement for nursing education in the EC was agreed as a three year course combining theoretical and practical work, and based on 12 years of basic and high school education. An annex has recently been added to the directives to secure implementation of the primary health care element in each EC country's programme.

Demographic changes, demands for more qualified professional workers at lower costs, changes in primary health care, and advances in medical treatment and technology will all increase the needs for both generalist registered nurses and those with specialist skills. Until now specialist education for nurses has varied widely in different European countries.

In some countries nurses have been educated in specific specialist areas such as psychiatry without having first had a general training. Specialist nurses of this kind are not allowed to work freely as nurses within the EC; the directive on free movement clearly states that it applies only to registered nurses with a generalist education.

In other countries nurses include one or two specialties within their general education, and in still other countries specialty education is always a form of further education after the general course has been completed. To preserve flexibility the European nurses' leaders decided that to comply with the directives specialty education should come after a general education. They also agreed that specialties should be widely interpreted in this context and should not be confined to the traditional fields. Further education programmes are now being developed to cover a wide range of topics.

61

Nursing research, too, is changing rapidly from small closed enclaves to a much more open setting. A group of European nurse researchers has been formed and a secretariat established. All over Europe nurses are working on the development of nursing performance standards and the registration of nursing data. This trend is further advanced in North America, but the systems developed there are closely related to the private health care system—and that is not what European nurses want.

One question still being discussed is whether the clinical responsibilities for nurses are comparable in the EC countries. The traditional role of nurses is different from one country to another, as is their position in the health hierarchy.

Coming changes in Europe, including the movement of people, businesses, and services, will stress the health sectors in every country; but at the same time there will be political pressure in every country for health care delivery to match the highest standards. Nurses expect these trends to lead to the roles of nurses in European countries becoming more closely comparable.

## Nurses's social challenges

Minimum employment standards for nurses as laid down in the International Labour Office document 149 have not yet been secured in all countries. The convention was agreed in 1977, and since then 30

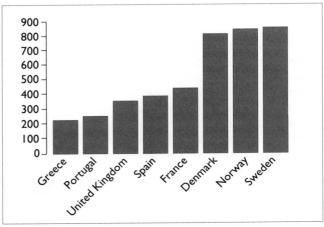

Number of qualified nurses per 100 000 population 1985

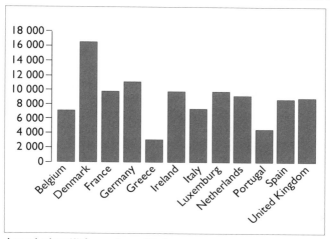

Annual salary (£) for newly qualified nurses

countries in the EC area have adopted it. Even though the WHO may provide technical assistance, including comparative statistics, for workforce planning in individual countries, reliable data are not yet available for Europe. At the moment the ILO is conducting a survey of nursing staff, but whether valid figures will emerge remains to be seen. The *Nursing Times* has collected some data on salaries (figure).[2]

The poor pay and working conditions for nurses in many countries have led to increasing unrest, with strikes in Britain and France. The tradition has been that nurses' salaries and the compensatory payments for night and Sunday duties have been lower than for other comparable groups such as teachers, police officers, and bank staff. This is partly a consequence of factors such as the close links between nursing and religious orders and partly because nursing is still mainly a profession for women. Nevertheless, in Europe attitudes to working women are changing rapidly and demands must be expected to grow for improvements in nurses' conditions.

The same trends are to be expected in the career structure. In many European countries the education of nurses has traditionally been a responsibility of the medical profession. This has already changed in some EC countries, in which nursing schools have nurse leadership. Animated discussions are continuing about whether nurses and nursing have their own identity and may make their own decisions in hospitals and in the primary health sector. Nurses claim this as a right in all sectors.

## The new challenges

The next 10 years will present many new challenges for the professions in Europe, and especially for the health professions. We do not expect the EC to issue directives on how to run hospitals or other health institutions, but we do expect minimum requirements to be set on health promotion activities and on health hazards. The full implementation of the social charter (in countries other than Britain) will also influence the health sector. Examples include the directives on the protection of pregnant women and women with small children and on workers with night shifts and changing duties.

The full implementation of coming directives on environmental matters will require nurses and doctors to take part in the discussions, since these questions are of great importance for health promotion and medical treatment.

As more citizens move from one country to another the whole health sector will need to become more flexible in its services and its educational systems. Many of the differences we know and live with today in the health sector will not be tolerated by the EC in the long run. Clearly, economic restraints will not allow limitless resources for health, but demands will continue to increase and this could lead to downward pricing of professional services. Doctors and nurses can fight this development, or we can choose to become the standard setters as advisers to the politicians. I prefer the second option.

1 World Health Organisation. Summary report. *European conference on nursing, Vienna, 21-24 June 1988*. Copenhagen: WHO Regional Office for Europe, 1988. (EUR/ICP/HSR 329(S).)
2 Seymour J. European round-up. *Nursing Times* 1990;**86**(48):38-41.

# Europe and nutrition: prospects for public health

MICHAEL O'CONNOR

After the second world war the major nutritional problems in Europe, if not the United Kingdom, arose from deficiencies of protein, minerals, and vitamins.[1] As western European economies recovered the problems became more those of overconsumption of nutrients such as fat, sugar, and salt. The problems are now ones of quality, not quantity, but the legacy of deprivation is still present. Much food policy is still geared towards producing large quantities of food and protecting the economic interests of farmers and food manufacturers rather than promoting healthy diets, protecting the environment, or even reflecting consumer demand.

## European dietary patterns

There are no standardised studies on consumption in Europe that can be used to produce compatible data on food or nutrient intake. It is possible, however, to use food balance sheets produced by the Food and Agriculture Organisation of the United Nations. These tables show the nature of the food supply and so may not fully represent what people are actually eating, but they provide a useful picture of trends in food consumption (figs 1 and 2; table).

Compared with just after the war Europeans now eat more food of animal origin and less of vegetable origin.[1] They eat every day the foods they used to eat on festive days. There are large regional variations. Mediterranean countries still derive a larger part of their energy from vegetable products than do northern European countries. The "Mediterranean diet" is believed to be healthier. Unfortunately, there are signs that these countries, and those in eastern Europe, are adopting unhealthy northern European diets.[2]

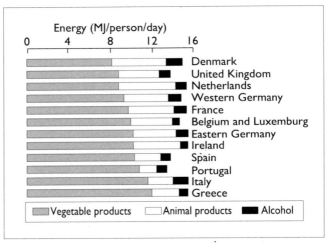

Figure 1—Total energy available per person per day from vegetable and animal products and from alcohol in European countries, 1979-81
Source: World Health Organisation

People in southern and eastern European countries suffer most from obesity, but as a whole the region compares favourably with other developed regions such as North America and Australasia.[3]

## Nutrition policy in the EC

In the context of current wider political debates some people may question the need for European nutrition policies. These are essential to maintain high standards because any product that is legally sold in one member state cannot be excluded from another state except for special reasons and on rare occasions. So in the absence of centrally agreed rules any member state's high standards—for example, on labelling, toxicology, or nutrient content—could be undermined by lower quality imports from elsewhere in the community. A more positive reason arises from the development of EC from simply a free trade area into a more rounded social and economic union.[4] While nutritional needs are biologically driven, diet is largely socially and economically determined.

One of the main reasons for the failure to develop integrated food and nutrition policies is that until the discussions at Maastricht are ratified the promotion of public health does not feature in the Treaty

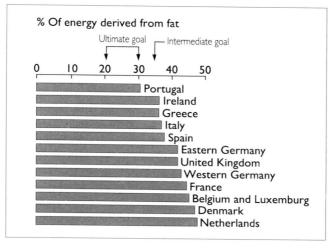

Figure 2—Estimated percentage of total energy derived from fat in some European countries
Source: World Health Organisation

of Rome, the legal basis for community action. Despite the lack of an explicit legal base EC policies do have an impact on health in, for example, food production and labelling, where trade concerns are involved.[5] In the World Health Organisation's charter, health takes precedence over trade; in the EC it has been the other way round and as a result the community has often trod blindly in matters of health.

The effects are clearly seen in the common agriculture policy. This fails to mention health as it is designed to secure production and meet the economic needs of farmers. The result is overproduction at vast cost to consumers and frequently in just those areas where in health terms we should be cutting back—for example, dairy products. A well known folly is the £900m spent each year by the EC on subsidising tobacco growing. Less well known is the £400m spent annually subsidising sales of butter to food producers.

There are proposals to revise the common agriculture policy.[6] Its vast costs, plus pressure from outside the EC to limit subsidies in the interests of fair trade, have made the current agreement untenable. Reform of the policy is not easy, and no government can afford to ignore the farming lobby, but the United Kingdom is supporting some reform. Ensuring that the common agriculture policy promotes health has not featured in the argument.

Intermediate and ultimate nutrient goals for Europe

| | Intermediate goals* | | Ultimate goals* |
|---|---|---|---|
| | General population | Group with high cardiovascular risk | |
| % Of total energy† derived from: | | | |
| Complex carbohydrates‡ | >40 | >45 | 45-55 |
| Protein | 12-13 | 12-13 | 12-13 |
| Sugar | 10 | 10 | 10 |
| Total fat | 35 | 30 | 20-30 |
| Saturated fat | 15 | 10 | 10 |
| Ratio of polyunsaturated:saturated fat | ≤0·5 | ≤1·0 | ≤1·0 |
| Dietary fibre (g/day)§ | 30 | >30 | >30 |
| Salt (g/day) | 7-8 | 5 | 5 |
| Cholesterol (mg/4·18 MJ) | | <100 | <100 |
| Water fluoride (mg/l) | 0·7-1·2 | 0·7-1·2 | 0·7-1·2 |

*Several ultimate and intermediate goals for the general population and the high risk group are the same: alcohol intake should be limited; iodine prophylaxis should be given when necessary; nutrient density should be increased; and body mass index should be 20-25 kg/m² (though this value is not necessarily appropriate for the developing world, where the average index may be 18 kg/m²).
†All values given refer to alcohol free total energy intakes.
‡These figures are implications of the other recommendations.
§Values are based on analytical methods that measure non-starch polysaccharide and enzyme resistant starch produced by food processing or cooking methods.

Another example of the domination of trade over health interests is the case of nutrition claims. The European Commission is currently drafting a directive on claims such as "low fat" and "high fibre." Its concern, however, is simply to secure fair trade rather than promote health. Recent drafts would allow nutrition claims if they were true in relation to similar products. Thus it would be acceptable to describe an intrinsically high fat product, such as a spread, as low fat if it is lower in fat than a similar brand. The United Kingdom Food Advisory Committee's recent report suggested basing definitions on an absolute rather than relative basis.[7] The Coronary Prevention Group and the International Heart Network have been urging a nutritional banding scheme as a base for defining claims.[8]

Nutrition banding is a system of describing the nutritional contents of foods by means of descriptors such as "high," "low," and "medium" for each nutrient in terms of the contribution it makes to the energy content of the food and the medical recommendations for the contribution that nutrient should make to an individual's energy intake if they wish to eat a healthy diet.

In general the European Commission has been reluctant to legislate on nutrition. It has limited itself to peripheral matters such as food additives, materials in contact with food, foods for particular nutritional uses, methods of preservation, inspection of premises, and enforcement of food law. Issues like food irradiation, labelling of permitted residues, and novel foods have not yet been agreed at a European level. In contrast, there are strict regulations governing agricultural products such as meat, milk, and eggs. Once again these are designed to promote trade rather than protect health. For example, the meat regulations apply only when meat is exported to another member state and not when it is for the home market.[9]

## The future

Europe's future diet will depend on many variables, including changes in public awareness, results of new scientific research, the response of the food industry, and the agricultural sector and government policies. The single market will develop, making trade easier, and larger enterprises will probably gain most. As a result, the market for food may become more concentrated in the hands

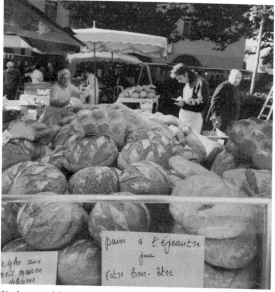

Endangered by the single market? The promotion of similar products throughout Europe may erode regional differences

of fewer producers. Multinational food companies may extend their operations across Europe and take a larger share of the market. Similar products, especially processed food with high added value and a range of nutrient values, may be promoted throughout Europe and this may erode regional differences (el, der, and le hamburger). Within countries a greater variety of foods may become available. Closer political union may make it easier to adopt international policies on food and nutrition.

British nutrition policy has recently taken important steps forward with the publication of dietary reference values by the Committee on the Medical Aspects of Food Policy[10] and the proposition of population nutrition targets in *The Health of the Nation*.[11] These are essential precursors to an integrated food and nutrition policy, but much remains to be done to find ways of helping and motivating people to choose a healthier diet.

## What is being done

It is unclear what will be done on nutrition as the whole future of EC health policy awaits the outcome of current deliberations on the implications of the Maastricht addition of public health to the Treaty of Rome. Before Maastricht the EC had declared 1995 to be European Year of Nutrition and they had drafted an action plan. Until we have an indication that they plan to be more radical we only have the old plans as a guide to how they see their role in promoting healthy nutrition. The draft targets were:

● To increase citizens' overall knowledge in the area of nutrition and awareness about the important relation between diet and health

● To increase the awareness of dietary habits that may lead to reducing disease related risk factors and enhancing health status and overall wellbeing

● To stimulate activities focusing on the nutritional needs of specific groups of the population

● To inform the general public of the effects and benefits, relative to quality and safety of foodstuffs, of community legislation

● To improve nutrition education in schools

● To encourage training in nutrition of health personnel

The size of the budget for these laudable objectives is not yet known, but latest rumours suggest it will be a paltry £8·5m. A wide range of activities is suggested, including:

● Promoting studies and investigations into the best ways of

protecting health and preventing disease by way of a balanced diet
- Disseminating knowledge about activities relating to food and health
- Encouraging greater consideration of nutritional and health aspects in other aspects of the community's activities
- Fostering awareness of hygiene in various stages of the food cycle
- Organising conferences and disseminating knowledge on the dangers of alcohol
- Promoting consumer understanding of food labels
- Stimulating activities focusing on the nutritional needs of elderly people
- Promoting training programmes on nutrition.

These measures are essentially passive. Like British policy they rely on health education rather than health promotion. At some levels there are signs that the community wishes to be more active in nutrition matters. For example, the commission has applied for membership of Codex Alimentarius, the world body that sets food standards. It will be unfortunate if the EC's voice is dominated by trade interests as are those of so many national delegations.

It is too soon to say how the EC will develop health policy following Maastricht but some positive developments seem possible:
- The EC's policy will be more coherent. Faced with a duty to make health protection a constituent part of other policies we may see improvements to policies such as those on agriculture and food labelling which have not previously been wholly conducive;
- The EC's policy may be more comprehensive. Previously the commission mounted measures such as Europe Against Cancer as a result of political initiatives. As such they were isolated and not part of any strategy. The money available depended heavily on whatever transitory political support was available. The commission's enthusiasm for these initiatives varied;
- The EC's policy will be better organised. As mentioned above it is possible that the health functions of the commission will be unified under a commissioner for health;
- The EC's policy will be better funded. Amid much publicity president of the commission, Jacque Delors, has sought a large increase in the budget to reflect the agreement at Maastricht. It is likely that some of this will find its way to health;
- The EC will take initiatives in promoting coordination of disease prevention policies;
- The EC will have a role in collaborating with the WHO.

## What should be done

Nearly half the deaths in people aged under 65 in Europe result from diseases to which diet makes an important contribution.[2] Improving the nutritional status of Europeans will require action by governments and voluntary bodies, food growers and processors, retailers and advertisers, the media and schools, and health professionals and individuals. Decisions should be taken at the lowest possible level. Each level should be responsible for the action best taken at that level. Policies should recognise and respect the diversity of dietary cultures across Europe. Governments, individually and acting collectively, should encourage and facilitate multisectoral and multidisciplinary working by establishing integrated food and nutrition policies.

It is easier to call for an integrated food and nutrition policy in the EC than to define one. Its development will depend on three factors. Firstly, it requires a sound scientific base. There is a continuing need for nutrition research, but a good deal is already known about what constitutes a healthy diet. Secondly, we need a strategic understanding of the interrelation of policies on production, trade, environment, consumerism, and general economics. Thirdly, we need to know more about health promotion policies that work. British nutrition policy is based heavily on health education; as such it fails to address the reasons why people do not always make a healthy choice despite a relatively high level of awareness. European policy must not fall into the same trap.

---

**Possible changes**
- Revised price support systems under the common agriculture policy
- Compulsory nutritional labelling
- Subsidies on foods for consumption by economically less advantaged regions and individuals
- Promotion of better training in nutrition for health professionals and caterers
- More medical and scientific research programmes
- Financial support for changes in manufacturing technology
- Public contract compliance on nutritional grounds
- A progressive tax on processed foods that would favour less processed products
- Controls on the promotion of foods containing large amounts of nutrients which are consumed in excess
- Regulations specifying minimum nutrient contents for staple foods

---

An integrated food and nutrition policy would reach into many areas under a new commissioner for health working alongside the commissioner for agriculture. Decisions need to be taken on priorities—a first step should be to agree on nutrient goals and priority areas for action. Target dates should be set, and should not preclude individual member states setting tougher targets. Once the EC has agreed its targets it should devise and implement policies to achieve them and establish systems to monitor progress. It should launch an immediate audit of all policies that have an impact on food and nutrition.

People cannot and should not be forced to eat a healthy diet, but society can contrive to make the healthy choice easier.

1 James WPT. *Healthy nutrition*. Copenhagen: WHO Regional Office for Europe, 1988:9.
2 Lang T, Miller M, Millstone E. *Final report of the study of the demand for differentiated food products in twelve member states of the European community*. Brussels: EC Consumer Policy Services, 1990.
3 Garrow JS. *Obesity and overweight*. London: Health Education Authority, 1991.
4 O'Connor M. Public health and the European community. *Health Education Journal* 1992;**50**: 200-3.
5 Richards T. 1992 and all that. *BMJ* 1991;**303**:1319-22.
6 Commission of the European Communities. *The development and future of the common agricultural policy. Green Europe*. Brussels: Commission of the European Communities, 1991.
7 Food Advisory Committee. *Food advisory committee report on its review of food labelling and advertising*. London: HMSO, 1991.
8 Coronary Prevention Group. *Nutrition banding: a scientific system for labelling the nutrient content of foods*. London: Coronary Prevention Group, 1990.
9 ECAS. EC non-policy on food and health. *The European Citizen* 1991 September.
10 Committee on Medical Aspects of Food Policy. *Dietary reference values for food energy and nutrients for the United Kingdom*. London: HMSO, 1991.
11 Secretary of State for Health. *The health of the nation*. London: HMSO, 1991. (Cm 1523.)

# Europe and tobacco

NICK BOSANQUET

Europe, with the highest per capita consumption levels for manufactured cigarettes of any of the six World Health Organisation regions, faces an immediate and major challenge in meeting WHO targets that a minimum of 80% of the population should be non-smokers and tobacco consumption should be 50% lower by 1995.[1] The European Community's policy has gained momentum, but mainly in relation to specific issues of advertising and labelling. Within some countries there have been some hopeful changes in policy—but there is not yet the commitment to a radical strategy which could alone secure progress towards WHO targets.

There has been some reduction in the number of people smoking since the 1960s, but smoking rates among younger Europeans remain far higher than in the United States. Further growth in mortality from tobacco related disease has slowed down in EC countries, but not enough has been done, apart from the United Kingdom and Ireland, to reduce the likely toll. Policy too is much less broadly based or coherent than might appear from the occasional high points. The EC has seen spasmodic attention from commissioners interspersed with long periods of sub-committee inertia.

Outside the United Kingdom and Scandinavia there is little consistent information about trends in smoking. The late 1980s are much better documented, partly through the commission's own efforts in developing surveys but also because of new research in France. Figures 1 and 2 show the basic data from the EC surveys.[2]

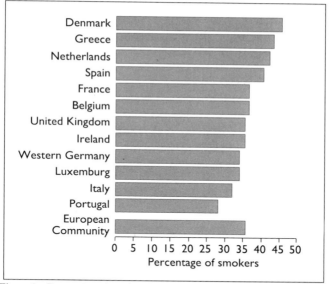

Figure 1 — Proportion of smokers in European Community countries, 1989

## Smoking rates

Overall smoking rates might seem reassuringly low with the community rate at 36%. This average is brought down, however, by the low rates of smoking among women in southern Europe, rates that are likely to rise over the next 10 years without strong policy initiative. For France the overall rate is affected by the low proportion of smokers among older men, which reflects the record up to the 1950s of relatively light smoking in France.

In many ways smoking rates for the under 40s are a much more telling indication of change and here the position is far less reassuring. The 25-39 age group should show a high demand for health where decisions can affect life expectancy. Smoking rates in Greece and Spain are in line with national stereotypes, but high rates of smoking are also found in northern Europe. Smoking rates for women in this younger age group are now as high or higher than for men. Fifty per cent of women in Spain aged 25-39, 49% in Denmark, and 43% in Italy are smokers, showing high levels of smoking at the age women are most likely to be pregnant. Reductions in smoking within the EC have been concentrated among older men. Smoking would seem to

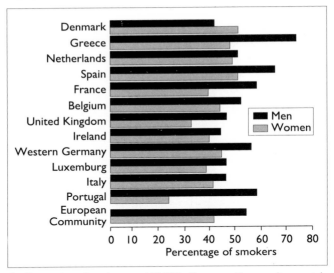

Figure 2—Proportion of smokers aged 25-39 in European Community countries

have increased recently among women in most EC countries and may well increase further as incomes rise.

In the United States and the United Kingdom specific groups gave a strong lead towards smoking cessation and more general changes in habit came about through a diffusion process. Doctors stopped smoking and were followed by other middle class groups.[3] By the late 1950s smoking had reduced among British doctors. There are few signs of this diffusion process at work across the EC (table). British doctors are unique in their rejection of the habit, with only 10% now smoking. In Spain and Italy higher proportions of doctors smoke than of the population as a whole. Smoking rates among teachers are a more hopeful indication.

New data from France about changes in cigarette consumption over time illustrate the size of the problem.[4] Tobacco sold in the form of cigarettes rose from 54 000 tons in 1965 to 95 000 tons in 1986, an increase of 76% over a period in which the adult population rose by 19%. Smoking remains high among young people and has risen among younger women.

## Costs of smoking

Survey results from the EC as a whole cast some doubt on the

Percentage of smokers in the European Community

|  | General medical practitioners | Teachers | Whole population |
|---|---|---|---|
| Belgium | 28 | 17 | 36 |
| Denmark | 38 | 34 | 45 |
| West Germany | 24 | 22 | 34 |
| Greece | 39 | 30 | 43 |
| Spain | 44 | 34 | 40 |
| France | 31 | 16 | 36 |
| Ireland | 20 | 15 | 34 |
| Italy | 41 | 36 | 32 |
| Luxemburg | 36 | 17 | 34 |
| Netherlands | 29 | 24 | 42 |
| Portugal | 39 | 21 | 28 |
| United Kingdom | 10 | 12 | 35 |
| European Community | 36 | 26 | 36 |

Source: Commission of the European Communities, 1989[2].

stereotype of the heavy smoking, happy go lucky south as against the health conscious north. Smoking is least common in Portugal, and German smokers are least likely to want to give up. Smoking rates in the north are particularly disquieting given the strength of the price disincentives. Forty five per cent of Danes smoke and pay 3.16 ecu for a packet of 20 (1986 prices), while 40% of Spaniards smoke and pay only 0.31 ecu a packet. Prices of cigarettes remained quite low throughout most of the EC. In the late 1980s only three member states had prices above 2 ecu (£1.40) a pack—the United Kingdom, Ireland and Denmark. There were four low price countries—Greece, Spain, France, and Portugal—where the price per pack was £1 or less; Benelux, western Germany, and Italy (all with high real incomes) were in the middle band.

Detailed evidence is available from the United States on costs of smoking and gains from abstention. As a result of the antismoking campaign, the Surgeon General estimated 789 000 deaths were postponed during 1964-85, 112 000 in 1985 alone. The average increase in life expectancy was 21 years.[5] The main forecast for Europe is a very broad one for the whole WHO area. It suggests that deaths from smoking related disease would increase from 0·8m in 1988 to 2m in 2025. Some of the increase is the result of demographic effects and the rising incidence of smoking in Russia and eastern Europe.[6] Increases within the EC may be less extreme. There was a 25% rise in mortality from lung cancer in France and Germany in the

77

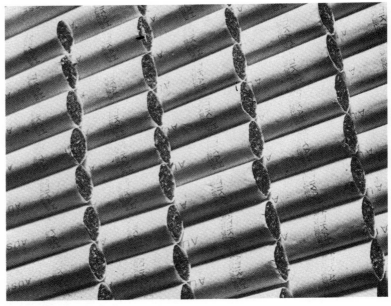

"Atikah Cigarettes" by Katt Both, 1931.

1980s.[7] This increase may not be so steep in the 1990s and beyond, but much will depend on policy in the immediate future. There will already be high inescapable costs from past decisions and past increases in smoking—but Europe could take actions that would prevent yet further growth in mortality and cost on into the twenty first century. What are the chances of an effective strategy?

## Approaches to a strategy on tobacco

Events over the past few months may have generated a false sense of optimism about the imminence of any such strategy. Much publicity has surrounded the initiative by the social affairs commissioner. As part of the EC's policy of extending the internal market, the commission has proposed a complete ban on advertising, apart from advertising in retail shops. The initial proposal will now be discussed by community health ministers. At present eight members seem to be in favour and four (Germany, Britain, Denmark, and Netherlands) against. The European Parliament will also give its view on the total ban. Some progress has been made through bans on television advertising. National pressure groups, such as ASH, are clearly gaining more influence.

The commission's original policy moves were on pricing, as part of fiscal harmonisation designed to produce similar rates of taxation across the internal market. This process has been dragging on over 20 years but received some new impetus in the late 1980s as policymakers became more aware of the health issue. Proposals in 1989 set target rates designed to increase taxation on cigarettes in southern Europe. However, such rates would have had perverse effects in reducing prices in the north. The council's new proposals simply set a minimum tax at 57% of the retail price, and a ratio of specific duty to total tax of at least 25%. These conditions are not onerous or even very clear in their implications for pricing, and in effect pricing will be left to the discretion of each national government.

The Europe Against Cancer campaign has led to a number of useful moves and has provided a framework for policy moves on tar yield, labelling, and advertising. Measures on labelling are designed to strengthen warnings and to extend them to products other than cigarettes. The EC is extending the British ban on Bandit, a new kind of smokeless tobacco. The EC has also set standards for reducing smoking in public places.

## Local activity

Effective action against smoking will depend on national governments in the 1990s as it is highly unlikely that the EC will be involved in actions which go beyond the symbolic and exemplary. EC actions can set a framework and stimulate local political activity but they do not seem likely to provide incentives powerful enough to bring about radical changes in smoking behaviour in the short term. Experience in Britain and the United States now gives some guidance on what an effective response might be. Any strategy for reducing smoking over a period as short as five years must make use of price incentives. A rise in the relative price of cigarettes is a powerful and effective means of reducing consumption. Recent simulations have shown that a 14% increase in the real price will lead to a fall in consumption of about 10%.[3] A doubling of the federal tax after 1982 was associated with a rapid decline in smoking in the United States and an increase in the state excise tax in California of 25 cents in 1988 led to an immediate decline of 19·4% in cigarette consumption. Reductions in smoking in the United Kingdom in the 1980s were concentrated in years when relative prices rose rapidly.

Authoritative statements about the health consequences of smoking from the government or from medical professions can influence the decision to smoke. The Royal College of Physicians in Britain and the Surgeon General's reports in the United States have influenced smoking behaviour. The Surgeon General has also created new issues, especially with his focus on passive smoking. Other measures, such as labelling, have a more minor impact, and even bans on advertising are less effective than price incentives.

There is some hope of a clearer and stronger strategy in France, where successive governments since 1988 have shown greater concern about the costs of smoking. France has also introduced new measures to restrict advertising and to limit smoking in public places, with accompanying fines. The issue seems, though, to get little attention in Germany, where discussion has tended to focus on the lighter types of policy measure involving peer group influence through sports stars and pop idols. There are now signs that Germany may adopt WHO targets.

Local political activity has increased and there have been some signs of coordination across the community, with European Bureau for Action on Smoking Prevention (BASP) playing a vital role in organising support for the directives. The United Kingdom has backed into a series of actions which have been relatively effective and it is now developing a strategy with possible targets of reducing smoking prevalence by about a third by 2000. The substantial increase in prices in the 1991 budget made a good start towards achieving these targets. Policymakers in Netherlands are also giving the issue greater attention. Ireland has a good record but is doing more.

## The outlook

Reductions in smoking have proved difficult in the EC area, and without strong policy initiatives rising real income would lead to a rise in smoking over the next decade. There are continuing conflicts of interest between agricultural policy and health issues, with community spending on subsidies to tobacco growers (£800m) still vastly greater than spending on the Europe Against Cancer campaign (£50m). The outlook for eastern Europe and Russia is even worse as there may be few competing forms of consumption over the next few

---

**Main EC initiatives**

**Europe Against Cancer programme**. The action plan covers:
- Cancer prevention
  - —Reducing tobacco consumption
  - —Research on nutrition and cancer
  - —Screening and diagnosis
- Information and health education
- Training of health professions
- Research on cancer

**Directive on labelling** (1989)—harmonises the content of labelling throughout the EC and provides for stronger health warnings

**Proposals for fiscal harmonisation** (1989)—now agreed by the Council of Ministers in terms of a minimum tax of 57% of the total price, leaving countries free to make their own pricing decisions

**Directives on tar yield** (1989)—limits permitted tar yield throughout the EC to 15 mg by the end of 1991 and 12 mg by the end of 1997. Greece has an exemption allowing higher yield till 2007

**Measures to reduce smoking in public places** with at least 50% of space in cafés and restaurants to be smoke free by 1992

**Ban on advertising in EC** (1991)

---

years and a 30 year lag in information about smoking. For wider Europe the WHO could strengthen its role. It has already set targets of reducing smoking prevalence to 20% by 1995 and produced a series of reports on a smoke free Europe as part of the Health for All by the Year 2000 programme.[1] The WHO could well be given a larger role. For example, it could produce annual reports on smoking in Europe based on cross national data. This would require special funding from national governments. The WHO would seem to be a better base for this reporting role than the European Commission.

Many countries in Europe face critical choices over the next two years in whether to adopt more active antismoking policies. On these decisions will depend whether the incidence of smoking related disease continues to rise. There could be an increased role for the BMA over this period in mobilising opinion against smoking doctors. A clearer stand by national medical associations could contribute to the more active policy phase. On this issue governments have followed opinion rather than led it.

1 World Health Organisation. *A 5 year action plan. Smoke free Europe.* Copenhagen: WHO, 1987.
2 Commission of the European Communities. *Smoking and the Wish to Stop.* EC Brussels 1989.
3 Bosanquet N, Trigg A. *A smoke free Europe in the year 2000: wishful thinking or realistic strategy?* (RHBNC/St Mary's Discussion Paper 4.) London: Carden Publications, 1991.

4 Hirsch A, Hill C, Frossart M, Tassin J-P, Pechabrien M. *Lutter contre le tabagisme.* Paris: La Documentation Francais, 1988.
5 Surgeon General. *Reducing the health consequences of smoking. 25 years of progress.* Washington: US Department of Health and Human Services, 1989.
6 Peto R. Total tobacco mortality. In: *1985 Estimates and 2025 Projections.* Copenhagen: World Health Organisation, 1988.
7 Department of Health. *The health of the nation.* London: HMSO, 1991. (Cm 1523.)

# Alcohol and drugs

MICHAEL FARRELL, JOHN STRANG

There has been an extraordinary diversity of substance problems in Europe, mirroring historical, cultural, religious, and political differences. The nature and extent of the problems associated with substance use vary, as do the moral, medical, social, and scientific responses.

In northern Europe people have drunk spirits, leading to a pattern of intermittent and explosive drunkenness, while in the south wine drinking has been integrated into a way of life with little public drunkenness and high risks of liver cirrhosis. In between there has been a belt of beer drinkers in Germany, the low countries, and Britain. The north has favoured Alcoholics Anonymous and fostered the temperance movement, while in France moderation was defined until comparatively recently as not more than a litre of wine a day.

A myriad of groups and organisations are involved in alcohol and drug policy in Europe, but the lack of a health directorate has rendered much of the data and issues impenetrable. Data need to be collated on a community wide basis. The Maastricht summit has committed the EC to some responsibility for health,[1] and drugs have been incorporated in the remit that will take effect in 1993.

## Alcohol

The rates of alcohol consumption and alcohol related problems vary greatly. Rates of consumption are higher in southern Europe. A consensus has developed among policy makers that the level of alcohol related problems in a society reflects the level of consumption,[23] which

83

is affected by cost and availability.[4] Traditionally, the northern European states have imposed higher levels of taxation and restricted availability. These are the countries which have invested more in medical and social research on alcohol and alcohol related problems and taken the problems more seriously by developing prevention and treatment programmes. Despite such polarities France has reduced consumption from 17·3 litres of 100% alcohol a head in 1970 to 13·2 litres a head in 1989,[4] and Italy has shown an even more dramatic reduction, from 16 litres to 9·7 litres a head between 1970 and 1989. Meanwhile, some of the countries with a low consumption have moved up—for instance, the United Kingdom moved from 5·3 to 7·3 litres a head between 1970 and 1989.[4]

*Taxation*

McGuinness has reviewed the impact of proposed EC legislation on alcohol consumption in the United Kingdom.[5] The right of individual countries to determine their own policy for controlling alcohol consumption and to modify it in the light of the rising incidence of alcohol related mortality and morbidity encapsulate some of the difficulties of European integration.[6] The proposed legislative change aims to introduce the single internal market to remove trade barriers. The community wants to standardise the legislation on the production, packaging, and presentation for sale of goods, and it is in this remit that standardised health warning labels and standard measures may be introduced on alcohol and tobacco products.

The original discussion of the single internal market and fiscal harmonisation failed to recognise the important role of alcohol taxation as an element of health policy. It was originally proposed to have a single rate of duty for each product group in all member states, but after considerable protest the European Commission relented to allow a 10% range to take greater account of the health aspects of alcohol consumption. According to McGuinness this fundamentally conceded the connection between alcohol taxation and health.[5] Having moved down this path the commission has now stated that it will allow each country to determine its own level of taxation on substances that may influence the nation's health.[7]

In the original discussion the acceptance of differential rates of taxation was viewed as a transitional arrangement where ideally countries would evolve to a position of equalisation. Countries with high tax rates may move down to come in line with other member states. The free flow of low cost alcohol across borders is likely to have marginal effect on national consumption rates in the United Kingdom but may pose problems for other countries.

*Consumption and morbidity*

A limited amount of collated data exists on European morbidity and mortality related to alcohol consumption. The table shows the most recent reports on national rates of alcohol consumption. The most graphic representation of the relation between alcohol consumption and death rates from cirrhosis of the liver in the mid-1970s represents the crude polarisation of consumption between northern and southern Europe (fig).[8] Governments face continuing political difficulties when reconciling the conflicting needs of the alcohol industry and revenue collection on the one hand and the needs of the general health of the population on the other hand. Some degree of compromise has been established but it is not clear how individual governments will fare in a larger Europe against a powerful multi-national corporate lobby pushing the health issues of alcohol further down the political agenda.

A range of laws deal with the consequences of alcohol consumption, such as public order laws, drinking and driving laws, and laws on the medical fitness to drive.[6] Some of these laws are coming under EC scrutiny.

*Production, distribution, and promotion*

The Scandinavian countries have traditionally been the most

Alcohol consumption per head of population in the European Community (excluding Luxemburg)

| | Litres of 100% alcohol per head | |
|---|---|---|
| | 1970 | 1989 |
| Belgium | 9·6 | 9·8 |
| Denmark | 7·1 | 9·6 |
| France | 17·3 | 13·2 |
| Greece* | 5·3 | 5·5 |
| Republic of Ireland | 5·9 | 5·8 |
| Italy | 16·0 | 9·7 |
| Netherlands | 5·5 | 8·1 |
| Portugal | 9·8 | 10·2 |
| Spain | 12·1 | 11·0 |
| Western Germany | 12·1 | 12·2 |
| United Kingdom | 5·3 | 7·3 |

*Beer and wine.

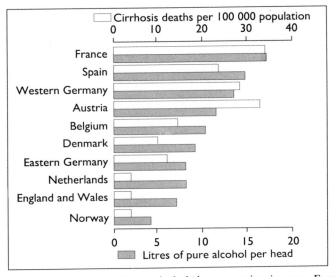

Deaths from cirrhosis of the liver and alcohol consumption in some European countries, mid-1970s

stringent controllers of production and distribution. Alcohol was rationed in Sweden at one time, and while an interesting case may be made for such an approach on health grounds it is clearly now a politically and socially unacceptable control strategy. The Scandinavian countries continue to have state owned production and distribution enterprises. Eastern European countries such as Poland, Czechoslovakia, and Bulgaria have successful state owned alcohol industries. The changes taking place in many eastern European countries have important implications for the balance between more restrictive alcohol control policies and the broader social liberalisation policies of the new market economies.

The Nordic countries, Switzerland, and France now ban alcohol advertising on public broadcast systems, and all countries have specific guidelines controlling the promotion of alcohol in public broadcasting. A fierce debate has raged on the imposition of controls banning the promotion of tobacco, and a similar move may occur with alcohol. The United Kingdom government continues to be one of the strongest advocates of voluntary agreements rather than imposed legislation.

Other areas of control are licensing laws, distribution laws, and laws on the advertising and promotion of alcohol products. More recently an EC initiative has made proposals for the labelling of alcohol products.

## Drugs

Although the introduction of the single market may loosen internal controls on alcohol consumption in Europe, the problem of illicit drugs has been viewed much more from the perspective of the loss of border controls and the impact that this may have on the supply of

---

**European organisations concerned with drug policy**

**United Nations**

The United Nations international drug control programme is involved in ratifying international drug control treaties that include Europe as part of its global responsibilities. Most countries have drug control policies ratified by the United Nations.

**Council of Europe**

The Council of Europe, established in 1947, has a remit to promote human rights through the European Court of Human Rights in Strasburg. It consists of 24 member states. The Pompidou Group was established in 1972 as a subsection of the council; its work has focused on attempts to develop epidemiological work on drugs in Europe.

**European Community**

The European Council (distinct from the Council of Europe) has agreed on the need for a coherent and effective drug control policy at a European level. Within the European Commission President Mitterand of France proposed the establishment of the European Committee to Combat Drugs, which started in 1989 and has advised the European Council that there was a need for a special emphasis on reducing the demand for drugs. It is proposed that this group should establish a European drugs monitoring centre to coordinate information on a Europe wide basis. The ad hoc "Group Toxicomanie" has a leaning towards health issues; and there is a planning group of the European Community's interior and justice ministers, which was originally established to fight terrorism but has incorporated the responsibility of drug enforcement into its remit.

**World Health Organisation**

The European office of the World Health Organisation's substance abuse programme aims, like the other organisations, to facilitate coordination and cooperation and is likely to have an important role in forging links between the EC and other European countries.

---

drugs—for example, from the newly established eastern European or Balkan route. Enforcement agencies are worried about the abolition of frontier borders and speculate that there will be increased ease of drug movement within and between countries once the outer European border has been crossed.

The diversity of approaches to substance problems is more extreme in the illicit drug field. The data on alcohol related problems seem to be limited, but the data on drug related problems are even more scarce. Because of the illicit nature of drug use the figures provided for the prevalence of use of opiates, stimulants, and other drugs are not far removed from guesswork. The 1980s saw Europe flooded with south west Asian heroin[9] and a rapid rise in the incidence and prevalence of opiate dependence.[10] This unfortunately coincided with the introduction of HIV to Europe. HIV has made manifest what otherwise could have remained an underrecognised problem and has placed great strain on health care, social welfare, and criminal justice systems.[11]

The north-south divide has curious parallels in the prevalence of HIV among intravenous drug users, with the Mediterranean countries of Italy, Spain, and France experiencing a much larger problem than their northern counterparts. There is no satisfactory explanation of the difference, but the variation in HIV prevalence may be best explained by the difference of time in the original introduction of HIV to the different countries. After the initial dramatic epidemic, recent figures suggest a levelling off since the second half of 1990 in the number of patients newly diagnosed as having AIDS.[10]

The World Health Organisation has just completed an inventory of drug problems in western and eastern Europe, which provides a collated overview of European problems but faces the inherent problem of any estimate of the prevalence of illicit behaviour. The changing situation in eastern Europe has resulted in increased availability of illicit drugs, and there are early reports of a considerable spread of HIV among Polish drug users.

### Treatment

A reasonable estimate of opiate use among different European countries would be 1%, excluding the Scandinavian countries, which seem to have a lower rate.[12] There is a definite disparity in the service response. The expansion of drug services in European countries has been driven by the increased prevalence of drug problems and by the public health implications of HIV. These services range from low threshold methadone programmes to residential rehabilitation treatment programmes. Netherlands has relied on a harm reduction model with methadone maintenance and low threshold methadone programmes; the British programme has relied on shorter term use of methadone with a mixed range of community and residential treatment programmes. France and Germany are estimated to have no more than 100 to 200 drug users receiving methadone and rely on abstinence in patient or residential treatment models. There is little evidence to correlate levels of treatment with reduced rates of HIV infection. This variation in treatment may cause drug users to migrate. The Netherlands and the United Kingdom have reported numbers of migrant addicts. This has important public health implications.

*Availability of needles and syringes*

The United Kingdom, Netherlands, and Switzerland have active needle exchange programmes in an attempt to limit the spread of HIV. Although Italy has had availability of injecting equipment through shops and pharmacies throughout the '80s, HIV has spread among addicts who inject themselves. Germany, France, and Belgium have relied more on the promotion of syringe cleaning techniques but also have retail outlets.

*Drug legislation*

The role of drug legislation and enforcement strategies has been critically reviewed in the past few years.[13] The link holding European legislation together is that it has been ratified by the 1961 United Nations convention, but different countries perceive the role of the law in differing ways.[14] For example, in Netherlands, although possession of drugs for personal use remains an offence, the law is rarely applied. It remains to be seen if such ad hoc arrangements will continue or if there will be pressure to harmonise implementation of

---

**Helpful target**

The adoption throughout Europe of the World Health Organisation's Health for All by the Year 2000 targets for reducing alcohol and drug consumption and containing the spread of HIV would be an important step in implementing effective public health strategies.

---

the law. It is estimated that 30% of the European prison population has a drug dependence problem.[11] With the advent of HIV and high rates of HIV in some European prisons there is pressure for a radical overhaul of the role of the criminal justice system in the response to drug problems in society.[15] Most European countries are moving towards a reliance on the treatment system but there is clearly a limit to this kind of response.

# Research

The EC has developed concerted action programmes to facilitate increased coordination and communication between researchers. The AIDS programme has included some drugs research, but there is a need for better research coordination on substance misuse and the World Health Organisation's Europe office has initiated a project to compile an inventory of European drug and alcohol research centres as the first step towards improving communications and collaboration.

We thank Tony McGuiness of the Institute of Alcohol Studies, Professor Griffith Edwards of the National Addiction Centre, and John Witton of the Institute for the Study of Drug Dependence for advice and information.

1 Waldegrave W. The health of Europe. *BMJ* 1992;**304**:56.
2 Royal College of Psychiatrists. *Alcohol—our favourite drug.* London: Tavistock, 1986.
3 Bruun K, Edwards G, Lummio M, Makela K, Pan L, Popham RE, *et al. Alcohol control policies in public health perspective.* Helsinki: Finnish Foundation for Alcohol Studies, 1975.
4 The Brewers Society. *Statistical handbook.* London: Brewing Publications, 1990.
5 McGuiness AJ. *Alcohol taxation and the European community.* London: Institute of Alcohol Studies, 1991.
6 Walsh D. *Alcohol related medico-social problems and their prevention.* Copenhagen: World Health Organisation, 1982. (*Public health in Europe No 17.*)
7 Amended proposal for a council directive on the approximation of the rate of excise duty on alcoholic beverages and on the alcohol contained in other products. *Official Journal of the European Communities* No 1990 January 18;**33**:12 (C12).
8 Office of Health Economics. *Alcohol—reducing the harm.* London: OHE, 1981.
9 Stimson G. The war on heroin: British policy and the international trade in illicit drugs. In: Dorn N, South N, eds. *A land fit for heroin.* London: Macmillan, 1987.
10 European Centre for Epidemiological Monitoring of AIDS. *Quarterly report no 30.* Paris: The Centre, 1991.
11 Harding T. *HIV/AIDS in European prisons.* Geneva: University Institute of Legal Medicine, 1990.
12 Council of Europe. *Multicity study of drug misuse.* Strasburg: Council of Europe, 1987.
13 Nadelman E. Drug prohibition in the United States: costs, consequences, and alternatives. *Science* 1989;**245**:939-46.
14 Leroy B. *The community of twelve and drug demand. Comparative study of legislations and judicial practice.* Brussels: Commission of the European Community, 1991.
15 Farrell M, Strang J. Drugs, HIV, and prisons: time to rethink current policies. *BMJ* 1991;**302**:1477-8.

# Prescribing in Europe — forces for change

DAVID TAYLOR

Legislation existing in or planned by the EC already affects the pharmaceutical sector in a wide variety of ways (box). It relates not only to how medicines are licensed, priced, labelled, and distributed but also to how they are manufactured and how clinical trials may properly be conducted.[1 2] Ultimately, every aspect of supply, from the post marketing monitoring of drug safety to the funding of research, may be influenced more by decisions made in Brussels than those agreed in individual member states.

The development of the EC single market is primarily intended as an economic measure. In the context of pharmaceutical trading it also has the potential to bring about considerable changes in the differing medical cultures of the EC's member states, influencing both the prescribing rights of the community's 600 000 practising doctors and the access to treatment of many of its 350 million citizens.

This chapter examines the extent of and reasons for the existing variations in consumption of medicines in Europe and the nature of the challenge facing those wishing to build a more unified EC medicines market. It then assesses the importance of current political debate about issues such as the costs of and access to medicines, safety of medicines, and the promotional standards of drug companies.

## Differences in use of medicines among EC states

All international comparisons may be subject to distorting factors. Nevertheless, the data presented in the figure and the table are broadly consistent with a range of sources.[3-5] They give an overview of differences in spending on medicines and dispensing volume in the

## Major EC pharmaceutical initiatives

| | |
|---|---|
| 1965 | First directive on human medicinal products established a general framework for subsequent national and EC legislation. |
| 1975 | Second directive led to the establishment of the EC's Committee for Proprietary Medicinal Products in 1976. First EC licensing procedures thus established. |
| 1975-85 | Limited developments—for example, in 1983 a council recommendation introduced preclinical and clinical guidelines, and medicine information and data requirements were amended. |
| 1985 | The Delors white paper put forward 13 proposals relating to pharmaceuticals. |
| 1987 | The biotech and high tech directive established new means of authorising and protecting products that might not have patents. It established the first pan-EC arrangements for licensing certain types of medicine. |
| 1989 | The "transparency" directive, which came into force in January 1990, sought to ensure that national decisions on medicine pricing and reimbursement are fair and made on a visible basis. It laid down a framework for cooperation and information exchange and required the commission to present before January 1992 further proposals to eliminate distortions in the EC market. |
| 1991 | Directives on the rational use of drugs, affecting wholesaling, harmonisation of legal status, and labelling and package information are nearing adoption. Also, a directive on pharmaceutical advertising has been prepared: it affects matters such as financial inducements and the distribution of free samples to professionals as well as advertising to the public, but will not now prevent companies from sponsoring medical meetings. |
| Under consideration | Future systems for drug authorisation, which at first will probably involve three approaches: a European Medicines Agency will be established in an as yet undecided location to handle centralised applications; the commission's proposals on supplementary protection certificates for medicines patents are under consideration, along with suggested controls on homoeopathic medicines and international drug testing harmonisation; a consultation document on clinical trials, aimed at controlling fraudulent practices and raising ethical standards, is in circulation. There are no proposals yet on the control of postmarketing surveillance initiatives and allied marketing interventions other than those in the "future systems" package. |

EC. Key points about the European pharmaceutical market include:

(1) Overall, richer countries spend more of their gross national product on health than do poorer ones, and in cash terms will usually spend more on medicines. Yet less affluent countries like Greece and Portugal spend much more on pharmaceuticals relative to their total health budgets than do better off states of the community.

(2) On a country by country basis Denmark is an illustration of a nation that combines lower than average domestic pharmaceutical consumption and spending with high medicine prices. France, by contrast, has low prices but high domestic usage and high medicine costs per head. The proportion of Danish gross national product spent on medicines is half that in France.

(3) In general, the EC nations with the highest medicine prices at home also have the most successful foreign trade records (Netherlands is an exception) and the lowest volumes of domestic prescribing (Germany is an exception).

(4) In northern EC states, such as the United Kingdom, Denmark, and Germany, over the counter medicine sales account for nearly a fifth of the total value of the medicines market. In Portugal, France, and Italy over the counter medicines represent only 5-10% of sales. (In the United States the equivalent figure is around one third, which implies that the EC over the counter market will expand during the 1990's, particularly if charges for prescription medicines are extended.)

(5) The United Kingdom combines relatively modest domestic consumption of and spending on medicines with a strong balance of trade and unusually high research spending. Largely because of Department of Health controls introduced in the 1970s it has unusually low levels of domestic spending on pharmaceutical promotion. Overall, about 10% of all NHS pharmaceutical revenue goes on promotion; equivalent European figures are about 15-20%.

(6) All European governments are showing increasing interest in promoting value for money with regard to publicly financed use of pharmaceuticals. Some new measures may limit doctors' prescribing; others restrict patient access to publicly purchased drugs; and yet others inhibit companies' abilities to sell or promote certain products. But at the same time nations wish to maintain or increase pharmaceutical industry investment within their borders, particularly in view of the manufacturing plant rationalisations that a more unified EC market may encourage. These conflicting motives may lead to apparently paradoxical policy decisions.[6]

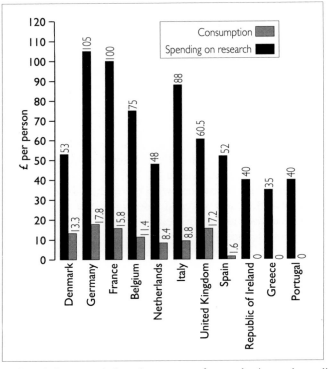

Consumption of pharmaceutical products at manufacturers' prices and spending on research, per head of population, 1989

Since 1989 there may have been some limited changes in the balance indicated in the table. For instance, government interventions in Germany has reduced some medicine prices there, while prices permitted in Italy for new products have been increased.[7] But the general position has remained surprisingly stable during the past three decades.

One important reason why this has been so is that the differences between European countries' prescribing patterns are based on deep rooted variations in medical culture and training rather than just the effects of contrasting price and profit controls for medicines.[8][9] Even so, such controls contribute to dramatic cost variations. In 1989 the Brussels based Bureau Européen des Unions de Consommateurs reported extreme illustrations of price distortion: Zyloric was 10 times

Costs and consumption of pharmaceuticals in EC countries, 1989

| Country | % Of gross domestic product spent on health services[16] | % Of health resources spent on pharmaceuticals | % Of gross domestic product spent on pharmaceuticals | Relative price of medicines, 1990 (EC=100)[17] | Implied volume of pharmaceutical consumption (UK=1) |
|---|---|---|---|---|---|
| Denmark | 6·3 | 6·8 | 0·47 | 129 | 0·8 |
| Germany | 8·2 | 10·6 | 0·87 | 128 | 1·6 |
| France | 8·7 | 10·8 | 0·94 | 72 | 2·7 |
| Belgium | 7·2 | 9·9 | 0·71 | 89 | 1·6 |
| Netherlands | 8·3 | 5·5 | 0·46 | 133 | 0·7 |
| Italy | 7·6 | 12·5 | 0·95 | 80 | 2·1 |
| United Kingdom | 5·8 | 11·5 | 0·67 | 117 | 1 |
| Spain | 6·3 | 13·8 | 0·87 | 73 | 1·4 |
| Republic of Ireland | 7·3 | 10·8 | 0·79 | 132 | 0·6 |
| Greece | 5·1 | 20·9 | 1·06 | 74 | 0·9 |
| Portugal | 6·3 | 23·6 | 1·48 | 68 | 1·1 |

Column 2 relates all pharmaceutical consumption (including over the counter drugs) valued at manufacturers' prices to all health care spending, public and private. In columns 1 and 3 gross domestic product is measured at market prices. The index of prices used is based on retail costings. Countries are ranked in order of gross domestic product per head, compared at 1989 exchange rates unadjusted for internal purchasing power variations. Population aged ⩾65 (high drug users) ranges from 11% in the Republic of Ireland to nearly 16% in Germany, United Kingdom, and Denmark.

95

more expensive in the United Kingdom than in Spain; Indocid 10 times more expensive in Netherlands than in Greece; and Microgynon eight times more expensive in Germany than in France.

The influence of professional traditions is reflected in the German acceptance of combination medicines, which British doctors would normally regard as unscientific and in some cases even unsafe. This partly accounts for the large number of branded medicines available in Germany.[7] The special cultural importance of issues relating to the heart is a possible reason why mild cardiac insufficiency and hypotension are regarded as diagnoses requiring treatment in Germany more frequently than in the United Kingdom.[9] Differing levels of promotional effort may also help to explain why, in the case of hypertension treatment, German doctors use diuretics more than their colleagues elsewhere in Europe. Similarly, British and German doctors often prescribe β blockers, whereas angiotensin converting enzyme inhibitors have gained a more dominant market position in Italy and France.[10]

In France patients apparently question their medical treatment less frequently than do patients in the United Kingdom. This may be one of the reasons why France now has the world's highest consumption of benzodiazepine sedatives and allied drugs.[11] In the United Kingdom this class of medicines is dispensed at nearly half the level recorded a decade or so ago. Whereas one French person in three took a hypnotic or tranquillising drug last year, the British figure is now probably less than one in ten.

For many years French doctors have also displayed a tendency to prescribe peripheral vasodilators. Next door in Italy, by contrast, use of tranquillisers has always been limited and peripheral vasodilators are less popular. Nevertheless, somatically expressed anxieties (and concerns about liver functioning in particular) have led to high sales of prescribed tonics and hepatic protectors.[8]

## The challenge facing Europe

The task facing agencies such as the European Commission in establishing a single European pharmaceutical market during the 1990s is daunting. It involves overcoming protectionist national structures which create waste and impair competition without— through pressing too hard for free trade and pharmaceutical cost savings—undermining companies' abilities to support research on medicines. European policy makers also need to try to ensure that over-enthusiastic moves to greater market unity do not cause the local values and preferences of patients and their physicians to be ignored.

For example, the perpetuation of wide price variations in medicine across Europe has obvious disadvantages, not the least being that it creates a sense of unfairness. The resultant practice of parallel importing* should help to level prices in time, to the extent that firms are free to adjust them. But it may promote lower than expected savings for health care systems or patients because of profit retention by middle men. And parallel importing does cut research based pharmaceutical companies' earnings.

Furthermore, too rapid transition to even pricing across Europe might have unfortunate effects on countries with low incomes or a high use of medicines, or both. Dismantling local price control schemes could encourage governments to use other methods of making savings in their pharmaceutical budgets—for instance, by raising charges to patients for medicines, which could cause real problems for poor communities.

Existing or proposed approaches to prescribing cost limitation in the EC include the following examples.

*Product by product price control:* This is the most common EC model, used in France, Belgium, Italy, Spain, Greece, and Portugal. In many cases it has been used to support local industry.[12] (Reference pricing, now being introduced in Germany and Netherlands, sets a basic price for entire drug classes. More expensive products in a given group have to be paid for directly by patients.)

*Company by company profit and cost control*—This is unique to the United Kingdom, where the Department of Health's pharmaceutical price regulation scheme has helped to achieve low promotion spending coupled with high research outlays. Details of the current scheme may, however, need to be modified in the face of the increasing Europeanisation of medicines trading in the United Kingdom.

*Positive and negative lists*—Examples of one or the other now exist in all EC nations. Their effect is either to restrict prescribing for patients of the public health care system to products approved on positive lists, or to block their access to medicines on negative ones. Controls over entry of products to such national lists—or local formularies—may limit the influence of the medical profession. (The introduction of

---

*Buying cheaply a given product in one country and selling it at the higher price in another. This affects little more than 1% of the value of trade in medicines in the EC overall but accounts for around 7% in the United Kingdom.

needs clauses in medicine licensing procedures, as in Norway, can be seen as a form of strict negative listing.)

*Patient copayment systems*—Charges may help restrict patient demand. Countries such as Belgium, Denmark, Greece, Italy, and Portugal vary the amount of prescription payment due inversely with the perceived value of the medicine. But high levels of exemptions to charges, as in the United Kingdom, decrease the impact of such systems. So too do back up private insurance systems to cover public service costs, as is most obvious in France.

*Generic or therapeutic substitution, or both*—Generic prescribing has been strongly encouraged in Denmark, Netherlands, the United Kingdom, and to a lesser extent Germany. Mandatory generic or therapeutic substitution (in which doctors' prescriptions are filled with products other than those actually specified) does not yet exist in the EC.

*Prescriber budgets*—Pioneered in the United Kingdom's fund-holding and indicative prescribing schemes, prescriber budgets are designed to increase prescribers' awareness of medicine prices without imposing rigid limitations on their judgment. Provided that the sums allocated are adequate and provision is made for unpredictable cost increases, this approach should combine the pursuit of cost restraint with respect for professional and consumer therapeutic choice.[6]

*Privatisation*—Encouraging the use of over the counter medicines and the private purchase of prescription drugs obviously shifts costs away from the public purse. The United Kingdom already has a sizable over the counter market, although no European country has—in relative terms—as great a volume of non-prescription sales as the United States. Denmark has a large over the counter market, coupled with private purchase of about a quarter of all prescribed medicines.

## Future threats and opportunities

Some commentators fear that attempts to create a single European market will break down medicine safety controls at a national level in a way that might benefit trade at the expense of consumer wellbeing.[13] The creation of the proposed new European Medicines Agency and allied bodies could reduce the importance of local institutions like the United Kingdom's Committee on the Safety of Medicines[14] and with it the influence of national medical establishments. This might make it easier for powerful industrial and allied interests to dominate regulatory activitives in the EC. As and when the agency comes into being in or around 1993 (the site is not yet decided, but it could be in Netherlands) care will have to be taken that its membership and working practices are as open and representative of informed public interests as possible.

It would be wrong to overstate, however, the risk of medicine safety standards being undermined by future EC arrangements for licensing. As suggested above a more potent threat to community wellbeing might stem from a weakening of medical control of public health care prescribing coupled with increasing pressures on consumers to pay directly for their medicines. Should this take place there will be a risk of depriving poorer people in Europe of access to effective care. This would be counterproductive in both social and financial terms, in that it could cause otherwise preventable ill health while undermining consumer confidence in existing provisions.

Those in government, the professions, and the pharmaceutical industry who are at present involved in lobbying to determine the structure of the future unified EC market should be aware of such dangers.[15] As is shown by the United Kingdom's record of keeping drug industry promotion spending down to about half the percentage of domestic turnover in countries such as France and Germany, there may be opportunities for reforms across the EC. But it would be foolhardy to interfere too quickly or too radically in structures that over the past 40 to 50 years have served public interests well. Compared, say, with eastern Europe's past record of low innovation and inadequate prescriber and patient access to drugs, that of the West is one thankfully to be preserved.

It is important to maintain the optimal amount of prescriber freedom and affordable access to medicines for all patients. Greater sensitivity to the price of medicines throughout the EC should not be gained at the expense of impairing society's ability to value effective treatment for everyone.

1 Sauer F. *The European community's pharmaceutical policy.* Brussels: Commission of the European Communities Directorate General for Internal Market and Industrial Affairs, 1990.
2 Barings Corporate Finance Healthcare. *The implications for the medical device and pharmaceutical industries of the EC's 1992 programme.* London: Baring Brothers, 1991.
3 Burstall ML. *1992 and the regulation of the pharmaceutical industry.* London: Institute of Economic Affairs, Health and Welfare Unit, 1990.
4 Association of the British Pharmaceutical Industry. *Pharma facts and figures.* London: ABPI, 1990.
5 Organisation for Economic Cooperation and Development. *Health care systems in transition.* Paris: OECD, 1990.
6 Taylor D, Maynard A. *Medicines, the NHS and Europe.* London and York: King's Fund Institute and Centre for Health Economics, 1990.

7  Smith T. Limited lists of drugs: lessons from abroad. *BMJ* 1985;**290**:532-4.
8  O'Brien B. *Patterns of European diagnoses and prescribing.* London: Office of Health Economics, 1984
9  Payer L. *Medicine and culture.* London: Goallancz, 1989.
10  Shearson Lehman Brothers. *Pharma pipelines.* London: Shearson Lehman Brothers, 1991.
11  Poll looks at French tranquilliser use. *Financial Times Pharmaceutical Business News* 1991; **157**:2.
12  Thomas LG. *Spare the rod and spoil the industry.* New York: Columbia University, 1989.
13  European drug regulation—anti-protectionism or consumer protection? (editorial). *Lancet* 1991;**337**:1571-2.
14  Griffin JP. Will the British Committee on Safety of Medicines be obsolete in 1993? *J R Coll Physicians* 1991;**25**:44.
15  Tross J. In: Thumbs down for commission action on pricing. *Scrip* 1991;**1629**: 4-5.
16  Schieber GJ, Poullier JP. International health spending: issues and trends. *Health Affairs* 1991; Spring:106-16.
17  Diener F. *Pharmazeutische Zeitung* 1990;**40**:2631-8.

# European research: back to pre-eminence?

RICHARD SMITH

Europe has an unequalled tradition in scientific research. Most of the important discoveries in science before 1900 were made by Europeans in Europe. Britain, France, Germany, Italy, Netherlands, and Switzerland had between them won 45% of all Nobel prizes from their inception until 1985—compared with the 39% won by Americans (table I).[1] Over those years, compared with the Americans, Europeans won twice as many Nobel prizes for chemistry, slightly more for physics, but fewer for physiology and medicine.

Although having strong traditions in research Britain, Germany, and France won most of their Nobel prizes in the early years of the century. The decline is most marked in Britain. Indeed, between 1986 and 1991 the United States won 22 prizes, the Germans nine, the Swiss three, the French two, and the British only one.[2] In terms of prizes per head of population from 1980-to 1991 the world order was the United States first followed by Germany, Sweden, Denmark, and then Switzerland.[2]

The hope in Europe is that the European Community and other bodies coordinating research across Europe will be able to produce greater collaboration and so eventually return Europe to the first place in science. In addition, research is vital for economic development, and better collaboration in research should increase the industrial competitiveness of Europe. But getting the countries of Europe to collaborate in research is by no means simple.

## Inputs and outputs in European research

Altogether the countries of the European Community spend about US$90 000m a year on research—considerably less than the

101

TABLE I – Nobel prizes by country, 1900-91

| | France | Germany | Italy | Netherlands | Switzerland | United Kingdom | Japan | United States | Rest | Total |
|---|---|---|---|---|---|---|---|---|---|---|
| **Physiology and Medicine** | | | | | | | | | | |
| 1901-1930 | 4 | 5 | 1 | 2 | 1 | 3 | 0 | 2 | 11 | 29 |
| 1930-1965 | 3 | 5 | 1 | 0 | 3 | 12 | 0 | 27 | 10 | 61 |
| 1966-1985 | 1 | 2 | 0 | 0 | 1 | 7 | 0 | 33 | 7 | 51 |
| 1986-1991 | 0 | 2 | 1 | 0 | 0 | 1 | 1 | 7 | 0 | 12 |
| **Chemistry** | | | | | | | | | | |
| 1901-1930 | 4 | 12 | 0 | 1 | 1 | 5 | 0 | 1 | 4 | 28 |
| 1930-1965 | 2 | 9 | 1 | 1 | 2 | 10 | 0 | 13 | 5 | 43 |
| 1966-1985 | 0 | 3 | 0 | 0 | 1 | 8 | 1 | 15 | 4 | 32 |
| 1986-1991 | 1 | 3 | 0 | 0 | 1 | 0 | 0 | 7 | 1 | 13 |
| **Physics** | | | | | | | | | | |
| 1901-1930 | 6 | 10 | 1 | 4 | 1 | 7 | 0 | 3 | 4 | 36 |
| 1930-1965 | 0 | 5 | 1 | 1 | 0 | 8 | 2 | 25 | 8 | 50 |
| 1966-1985 | 2 | 1 | 1 | 1 | 0 | 6 | 0 | 24 | 5 | 40 |
| 1986-1991 | 1 | 4 | 0 | 0 | 2 | 0 | 0 | 8 | 0 | 15 |
| **Total** | 24 | 61 | 7 | 10 | 13 | 67 | 4 | 165 | 59 | 395 |

$144 000m spent in the United States but more than the $57 000m spent in Japan (table II).[3] The expenditure per head of population ($201) is much less than that of both the United States ($582) and Japan ($469). The European countries spending the most on research are unsurprisingly those with the largest economies, with the Germans spending the most in absolute terms and the most per head of population ($431). Table II shows a clear divide in expenditure on research between the richer and poorer countries in Europe: Greece, Ireland, Portugal, and Spain all spend under $90 per head, whereas all the other countries spend over $170. Table III shows the growth (or in the cases of Ireland and Netherlands contraction) in expenditure on research by country for 1989: with an average expansion of 4·7% the EC is running ahead of growth in the United States (2·3%) but behind growth in Japan (9·1%).

Total expenditure on health research in the EC ($2045m) is less than a quarter of the expenditure in the United States, meaning that the Americans spend more than eight times as much per head on health research as the Europeans (table IV).[4] (The most surprising figure in the table is for Denmark, where Organisation for Economic Cooperation and Development data show that expenditure on health research has fallen from Kr 243m in 1986 to Kr 80m in 1990.)

How much do European countries have to show for their expendi-

TABLE II—Gross expenditure on research in European Community, United States, and Japan and expenditure per head of population, 1989

| Country | Expenditure on research (US$m) | Expenditure on research per head (US$) |
|---|---|---|
| Belgium | 2 059 | 208 |
| Denmark | 1 147 | 223 |
| France | 21 052 | 342 |
| Germany | 28 418 | 431 |
| Greece | 339 | 34 |
| Ireland | 268 | 73 |
| Italy | 12 095 | 173 |
| Netherlands | 4 412 | 297 |
| Portugal | 328 | 32 |
| Spain | 3 722 | 77 |
| United Kingdom | 18 485 | 323 |
| European Community total | 92 325 | 201 |
| United States | 144 820 | 582 |
| Japan | 57 740 | 469 |

TABLE III—Compound annual growth or contraction in gross expenditure on research for 1989

|  | Compound annual growth |
|---|---|
| Belgium | 2·3 |
| Denmark | 4·5 |
| France | 6·2 |
| Germany | 4·9 |
| Greece | 6·9 |
| Ireland | −0·7 |
| Italy | 4·8 |
| Netherlands | −0·3 |
| Portugal | 10·1 |
| Spain | 9·6 |
| United Kingdom | 3·7 |
| European Community average | 4·73 |
| United States | 2·3 |
| Japan | 9·1 |

TABLE IV—Total expenditure on health research for 1990 together with expenditure per head of population

|  | Total expenditure (US$m) | Expenditure per head (US$) |
|---|---|---|
| Belgium | 30 | 3 |
| Denmark | 13 | 2 |
| France | 494 | 9 |
| Germany | 498 | 8 |
| Greece | 12 | 1 |
| Ireland | 4 | 1 |
| Italy | 332 | 6 |
| Netherlands | 60 | 4 |
| Portugal | 6 | 1 |
| Spain | 144 | 4 |
| United Kingdom | 451 | 8 |
| European Community | 2044 | 4·27 |
| United States | 8572 | 34·46 |

ture on research? Science policy experts have various measures of "output," including numbers of publications, citations, patents applied for, and Nobel prizes. (A 300 page report on such data is currently being prepared for the European Commission.) Table V shows the number of patents applied for by nationals of the various

TABLE V—Total applications for patents filed by foreign nationals in the United States in 1988 together with number per 100 000 population

|  | Total patent applications | Patent applications per 100 000 population |
| --- | --- | --- |
| Belgium | 588 | 5·92 |
| Denmark | 535 | 10·42 |
| France | 4 902 | 8·73 |
| Germany | 12 493 | 20·15 |
| Greece | 29 | 0·29 |
| Ireland | 103 | 2·93 |
| Italy | 2 096 | 3·64 |
| Netherlands | 1 613 | 10·86 |
| Portugal | 7 | 0·07 |
| Spain | 231 | 0·59 |
| United Kingdom | 5 805 | 10·14 |
| European Community total | 28 402 | 8·72 |
| Japan | 29 613 | 24·05 |

European countries and Japan in the United States in 1989.[1] Together all the countries of the European Community applied for fewer patents than Japan alone, which suggests that the Japanese are much better than any European nation—except the Germans, who also had a high rate in terms of population—at turning scientific ideas into products.

Publication data are less easy to find for all European countries but figure 1 shows that the Swiss and the Swedes lead the world in numbers of scientific publications per head of the population.[5] Figure 2 shows world share of scientific publications, with the Americans contributing a massive 35%; the British, Germans, French, and Dutch between them contribute 23%.[6] When it come to citations the Americans dominate even more, accounting for 51% of citations, while the British, Germans, French, and Dutch account for 21% (fig 3). In clinical medicine the Americans produce 40% of publications and 54% of citations, while the British, Germans, French, and Dutch produce 27% of publications and 19·9% of citations.[6] An analysis of citations by subject shows that the French and Germans are both strong in chemistry, physics, and mathematics, while the British are strong in clinical medicine and biology and the Dutch in mathematics.[6] An analysis of trends in citations between 1983 and 1986 shows the world share of the Germans, British, and French is falling while that of the Dutch has stayed steady.[6]

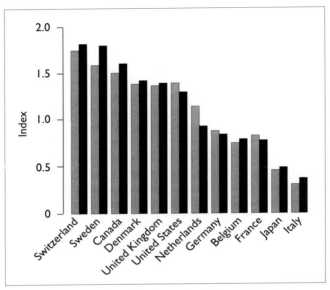

Figure 1—Number of scientific publications per head of population (various countries, situations 1977-9 and 1987) Comparison is with number of publications per head for the Netherlands in 1981, which is thus given the index of 1

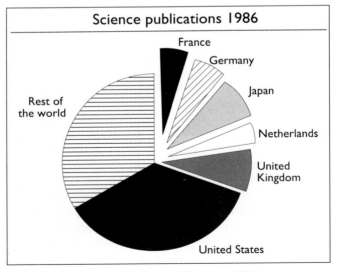

Figure 2—National shares of world science publications, 1986

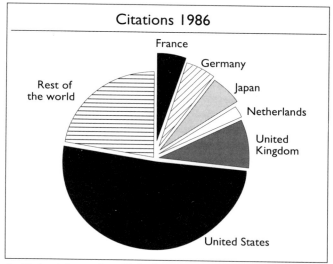

Figure 3—National shares of world citations, 1986

Generally these figures show that Europeans spend a lot on research, but not as much as their main competitors, and that they produce good results—but again not as impressive as their main competitors. The hope is that the European Community will eventually be able to produce a bigger bang for the research ecu by bringing the research efforts together.

## Networks of European research

The European Community is not the only organisation trying to bring scientists together in Europe. Science has always been an international activity, and many networks link scientists together across Europe. Many form personal links through travelling to international conferences, corresponding, and reading the same journals, and an increasing number are linked by electronic networks. There are, in addition, a host of societies covering most of the major scientific interests.

Despite these networks there is a need for larger organisations, and a good example is the Centre Européen de Recherche Nucléaire. It was founded in 1954 to bring European particle physicists together and give them the facilities to practise their expensive science. It effectively saved European high energy physics from extinction and

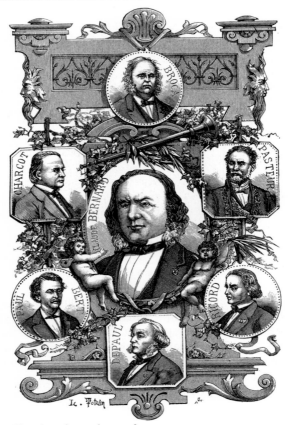

French genius on the wane?

showed that European countries could cooperate on a scientific endeavour that was beyond the means of individual countries. The European Molecular Biology Organisation was founded on a similar model in 1963.[7] The founders of the organisation, who included John Kendrew, the Nobel prize winning molecular biologist from Cambridge, were "deeply concerned that the initiative in molecular biology was by 1962 passing rapidly to the USA from Europe, where many of the early key discoveries had been made." They were "convinced that Europe could only play its accustomed role in the far reaching intellecutal movement that molecular biology represented if the individual countries pooled at least some of their national resources in this field of research." The private self governing organisation now has 700 molecular biologists as members and a laboratory in Heidelberg. It works by encouraging and funding interactions among European molecular biologists.

Another important grouping of European scientists is the European Science Foundation. The foundation has 56 member research councils, academies, and institutions from 20 countries. Funded by contributions from its members, the foundation "brings European scientists together to work on topics of common concern, to co-ordinate the use of expensive facilities, and to discover and define new endeavours that will benefit from a co-operative approach." Scientists like the foundation because — in contrast with the European Commission programme — it is led by scientists and academics and members can opt in or out of particular programmes: its menu is à la carte. But, as one observer of the foundation told me, "Its organisation is fantastically complex — only scientists could have created it."

Included within the European Science Foundation is a standing committee of the European Medical Research Councils that covers 13 national research councils. It has no budget, no sanctions, and only a small secretariat but allows the research councils to get together and discuss issues like training, the state of clinical research, data protection, and ethical issues.

Another important European body that is showing an increasing interest in research — particularly the ethical aspects — is the Council of Europe. Any interest in research is welcomed by the scientific community, but the proliferation of European bodies interested in research may mean that the energy that should come from strategically concentrating resources may be lost.

## Research and the EC

If any organisation in Europe can achieve widespread European cooperation in research that body is the European Commission. The European Community was born with two main aims — to prevent another war in Europe and to bring the countries of Europe together so that they could compete effectively with the United States and Japan. Research can contribute to both of these aims. In the early days research was conducted almost entirely in the subjects that were of particular interest to the community — coal, steel, and nuclear energy.[8] In the early '80s the community began programmes designed to coordinate research — the framework programmes — but it was the

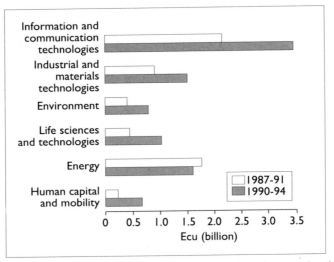

Figure 4—European Community expenditure on research under second and third framework programmes

Single European Act of 1987 that gave a real boost to research and development. That revision of the Treaty of Rome led to research and technological development being given the same status as economic and social policy. Figure 4 shows how funding has grown from the second research framework programme, which ran from 1987 to 1991, to the third, which runs from 1990 to 1994.

Because the Treaty of Rome did not cover health and biomedical research this has never been a large part of the community's research effort, but it is now growing. The programme is run by directorate general XII—the directorate for science, research, and development—and it began in 1978. At that time only three projects were supported, and the budget was 1·09m ecu.

The idea of the framework programmes, which began in 1984, is to bring researchers from different countries together to do largely precompetitive research. "The intention," says the commission, "is to deal only with projects that can be carried out more rationally, cost effectively and more efficiently at European level."[8] Research funds are thus largely devoted to coordination rather than funding particular projects, a point which some of those seeking grants have been slow to grasp.

The biomedical and health research programme (known as

BIOMED) is one of the smallest of the 15 research programmes being run by the commission—table VI shows all the programmes. BIOMED has a budget of 133m ecu, which is only 2·3% of the total research budget. The chief objective of BIOMED "is to contribute to improving the effectiveness of research and development in medicine and health in the member states, in particular through better coordination of their research and development activities, to applying their findings through community co-operation and to using available resources in common." Table VII shows how the scale of EC medical research has grown since its inception. It has grown exponentially at a time when most national research programmes have expanded little or not at all. The proportion of national research funds devoted to EC research is still tiny, but the present changing patterns suggest that eventually most research will be conducted on a European scale. The rapid growth of the European programme has, however, caused difficulties for the small numbers of staff who have overseen the programme since the beginning.

TABLE VI—European Community research and development third framework programme 1990 to 1994

| Programme | Ecu (millions)* | £ (millions) |
|---|---|---|
| Information technology and telecommunications: | | |
|    Information technology | 1352 | 942 |
|    Communication technology | 489 | 341 |
|    Telematics | 380 | 265 |
| Industrial and materials technologies: | | |
|    Industrial materials technology | 748 | 521 |
|    Measurement and testing | 140 | 98 |
| Environment: | | |
|    Environment | 414 | 289 |
|    Marine science and technology | 104 | 72 |
| Life sciences and technologies: | | |
|    Biotechnology | 164 | 111 |
|    Agriculture and agroindustrial research | 433 | 232 |
|    Biomedical and health research | 133 | 93 |
|    Science and technology for developing countries | 114 | 77 |
| Energy: | | |
|    Non-nuclear energies | 157 | 109 |
|    Nuclear fission safety | 199 | 139 |
|    Fusion | 458 | 319 |
| Human capital and mobility | 518 | 361 |
| Total | 5700 | 3972 |

*Central exchange rate mechanism: 1·435 ecu=£1.

111

TABLE VII—Growth in medical and health research in the European Community

| Programme | Duration | No of projects | No of national teams | Ecu (millions) |
|---|---|---|---|---|
| First | 1978-81 | 3 | 100 | 1·09 |
| Second | 1980-83 | 7 | 230 | 2·32 |
| Third | 1982-86 | 34 | 1400 | 13·3 |
| Fourth | 1987-91 | 140 | 4500 | 65 |
| Fifth | 1990-94 | ≥200 | ≥5000+ | 133 |

*Origins of a programme*

The way that a programme arises is complex and slow, and is summarised in figure 5. The proposal arises in the commission and is ultimately carried out by the commission, but it spends some two years going backwards and forwards between the commission, the parliament, and all three levels of the Council of Ministers. That is why applications are only now being processed for the framework programme that was due to begin in 1990. The complexity and slowness of the process is an important problem, but unfortunately the British blocked proposals to simplify and speed up the process at the EC summit meeting in Maastricht last year. The process of finalising a programme gives ample scope for political horsetrading, and substantial changes may be made. Thus Alain Pompidou, the Frenchman who is rapporteur of the research committee in the parliament, managed to have biomedical ethics included as a main target area in the programme.

The programme has four main target areas: prevention, care and health systems (21% of expenditure); major health problems and diseases of great socioeconomic impact (54%); human genome analysis (21%); and biomedical ethics (3·5%). The box shows the topics covered in the programme. The programme is particularly interested to encourage health services research, multidisciplinary teams where local skills are in short supply, clinical trials, targeted research where coordination is needed (for instance, research into AIDS or the human genome), and training. "In effect," says Gillian Breen, head of the international section at the Medical Research Council, "almost anything has a chance of getting funded."

Everything except the work on the human genome is supported primarily through concerted action contracts. These meet 100% of the costs of coordination and cover activities like organising meetings

112

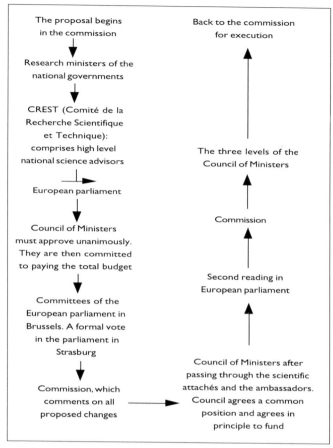

Figure 5—Long, slow journey through Europe of a proposal for a European Community research programme

and scientific support, distributing material and data, short term exchanges of staff, and dissemination of results. Shared cost contracts are for the human genome work and cover 50% of the full costs of the project or 100% of the marginal costs. These contracts are open to everybody and all organisations in the member states, but applications have to be made by partners from at least two member states. Austria, Finland, Norway, Sweden, Switzerland, and Turkey are all continuing an association with the programme and more countries are expected to join, with Czechoslovakia, Hungary, Ireland and Poland all now eligible.

### Approving projects

The system used for approving projects in the second framework was severely criticised by a group from York University appointed by the commission to evaluate the medical and health research programme.[9][10] The group said that many scientists in Europe knew nothing about the programme and did not know how to get grants from the commission; that the peer review system was below acceptable standards; and that the money would be better spent on a few centres of excellence rather than on paying people to coordinate with each other. The commission responded by improving its peer review systems.

The peer review system to be used in the third framework programme is currently being developed. The call for applications finally went out at the end of September 1991, and they were due in by the end of January 1992. Some 1900 applications were received, many more than for previous programmes. These are not full applications but outline proposals, and the commission aims to reduce them to about 250 in the next stage. The authors of these applications, which must come from more than one country, will then be invited to submit full proposals.

The outline proposals are about six to eight pages long and comprise one page summarising the current state of the proposed research subject; two pages on what is proposed; an explanation of why the application is being made through Brussels; a list of the participating teams; and a timetable and budget. These applications have been looked at by a series of panels consisting of 18 people (one from each country) divided into five disciplines: cell and molecular biology; physiology and clinical medicine; epidemiology and clinical trials; health services research; technology development and ethics. The panels have been put together from 750 names, nearly all proposed by the 18 countries, but they are anonymous—not even the Committee of an Advisory Nature on Biomedical and Health Research, the expert body which advises the secretariat running the programme, knows who individual panel members are.

The panels have scored the proposals on seven different criteria; scientific excellence and originality; relevance to the programme; transnational collaboration; the complementarity of the participating

---

### Scope of the BIOMED programme

BIOMED has four main target areas as follows:

Area 1—Development of coordinated research on prevention, care and health systems: 27·5 m ecu, 21% of the programme. Specific targets include: drugs, occupational health, biomedical technology, health services research.

Area 2—Major health problems and diseases of great socioeconomic impact: 72 m ecu including 25 m ecu for AIDS, 54% and 19% of the programme respectively. Specific targets include: AIDS, cancer, mental illness and neurological disease, cardiovascular disease, and aging and age related problems.

Area 3—Human genome analysis: 27·5 m ecu, 21% of the programme. Specific targets include: improvement of the genetic (linkage) map, physical mapping, DNA sequencing, data handling and databases, and technology development and applications of human genome analysis.

Area 4—Research on biomedical ethics: 4·6 m ecu, 3·5% of the programme. This will cover both ethical questions related to the programme and the evaluation of the social impact of the programme and the risks (including technological risks) which might be associated with it.

---

teams; the competence of the teams; the feasibility of doing the work within the three years available; and the potential for exploitation. The ethical and health and safety aspects of the proposals are also considered. The panels give a score to each of the proposals, which are then ranked and presented to the Committee of an Advisory Nature. The committee was presented with some 200 applications in category A with the recommendation that these all proceed to the next stage and some 1600 in category C with the recommendations that they would not be funded. At the end of the process about 100 projects can be funded.

In the next stage new subcommittees were formed, the members of which were not anonymous. There is one representative from each country with additions representing particular scientific interests. The subcommittees aim at matching the applications with the budget allocations. The Committee of an Advisory Nature met in June to make the final recommendations, but there will then be a second round of applications, with a closing date in January 1993.

*Top down and bottom up*

It is obviously tricky to fit together detailed instructions from above

115

about what should be in the programme with the applications coming from the scientists in Europe. The chance of all the best applications fitting into the preordained programme must be almost nil. Inevitably there have to be compromises on scientific quality in order to squeeze the applications into the various sectors. There are not, however, any priorities attached to the many parts of the programme, and the commission has been anxious to avoid such priorities—they might prove to be an impossible straitjacket.

Scientists are also inevitably suspicious of a funding process so dominated by political concerns. The politicians are prominent in deciding what should be in the programme, and then the peer review committees are structured to have one person from each country on each committee: it seems unlikely that those will be the best people that the community could produce to assess papers.

A final problem with the process is the shortage of staff to run the programme. It may seem strange to argue that there are too few bureaucrats in Brussels, but the 14 staff running the last 80m ecu programme were overstretched and the problems are likely to be worse with only 18 staff running a 133m ecu programme.

## Conclusion

Europe has in the past been pre-eminent in science and technology, but it has now lost that pre-eminence to the Americans and the Japanese. The standard and productivity of European science could almost certainly be improved by increasing collaboration among scientists in Europe. Various bodies exist to increase that collaboration, but the organisation best positioned to increase it dramatically is the European Community. Unfortunately, its processes for funding biomedical research are slow, tortuous, and muddy and need to be considerably improved before European nations will be willing to allow large parts of their research budgets to be spent through Europe. But that is surely what will need to happen in the end if European science is to be brought back to pre-eminence.

1 Advisory Board for the Research Councils, Royal Society, Economic and Social Research Council. *Evaluation of national performance in basic research*. London: ABRC, 1986.
2 Martin BR, Irvine J. The position of British science. *Nature 1992*;355:760.
3 Organisation for Economic Cooperation and Development. *Main science and technology indicators*. Paris: OECD, 1991.
4 Organisation for Economic Cooperation and Development. *Basic science and technology indicators*. Paris: OECD, 1991.

5 Van Heeringen A, Langendorff ANM. *Science and technology indicators.* Hague: Advisory Council for Science Policy, 1989.
6 Martin BR, Irvine J, Narin F, Sterritt C, Stevens KA. Recent trends in the output and impact of British science. *Science and Public Policy* 1990;**17**: 14-26.
7 European Molecular Biology Organisation. *European Molecular Biology Organisation 1964-1989.* Heidelberg: EMBO, 1989.
8 Commission of the European Communities. *EC research funding.* Brussels: EC 1990.
9 Maynard A, ed. *Evaluation of the fourth medical and health research programme.* Brussels: European Commission, 1990.
10 Richards T. European research. *BMJ* 1990;**301**:950.

# A common ethics for a common market?

SØREN HOLM

Inevitably the growing economic and political integration in Europe will lead to attempts to integrate the legal rules and the paralegal regulations, declarations, and statements that govern medical ethics. There have already been some moves in this direction.

The main institutions on the European scene are the Commission of the European Community, the European Parliament, the Council of Ministers of the European Community, and the Council of Europe. The last of these is a non-EC body of which all democratic states in the European region are members.

The Council of Europe has been the most active, through resolutions in its committee of ministers and its parliamentary assembly and through its standing committee of experts in bioethics. Medical ethical questions fall outside the scope of the Treaty of Rome unless they coincide with questions concerning consumer protection or other market related issues.[1] This explains the relatively limited involvement of the EC in the field. The Council of Ministers has, however, recently issued a series of statements on AIDS. This anticipates the probable inclusion of health and social issues in the coming treaty on European union.

All these official bodies issue statements, declarations, and directives with widely different legal status.* They are supplemented by powerful but less official bodies like the Standing Committee of Doctors of the EC and the Roman Catholic Congregation for the Doctrine of Faith. Researchers interested in medical ethics have also

---

*Only directives issued by the European Commission or the Council of Ministers have legal force in the member countries of the EC. The European Parliament can issue resolutions, but these have no immediate legal force. Recommendations and resolutions of the Council of Europe have legal force only in so far as they influence the legislatures in the member countries.

formed the European Society for Philosophy of Medicine and Health Care and the European Association of Centres of Medical Ethics.

## When in doubt form a committee

A consistent feature of the debates about medical ethics in Europe has been that governments have felt a need to establish investigative committees, commissions, or councils to discuss and clarify the problems. Some of these bodies have been able to reach agreement on specific policy proposals whereas others have been divided. Most have been single issue ad hoc bodies, but some countries—for example, France and Denmark—have established permanent ethical councils.[2][3]

Apart from their stated objectives of fact finding and policy making such commissions fulfil a variety of other political purposes.[4] So it is likely that the same approach will be chosen at the European level, initially in the form of ad hoc committees and perhaps later as permanent organisations. But it is doubtful that such commissions can represent the full width of the cultural diversity in the EC. The Glover working party on reproductive technologies authorised by the commission managed to reach a consensus, but its seven members did not represent the full diversity of the EC.[5]

## Abortion, IVF, and embryo research

Almost every European country has had its own commission on abortion, in vitro fertilisation, and embryo research, and these have been supplemented by the Congregation of the Doctrine of Faith,[6] the Glover working party,[5] and by the standing committee of experts in bioethics (CAHBI).[7] The guidelines proposed vary from the relatively liberal to the conservative. The resulting legislation is also divergent,[8] and it is difficult to see how a common European policy could be established. The commission took no action after the Glover report and it is unlikely that any action will be taken.

## Genetic screening

European guidelines for the use of genetic information do not exist, although the EC has allocated resources for research on the ethical issues created by the use of genetic information in the general genome research programme.[9] During the planning phase of this programme

the emphasis was changed from "prediction" to "medical importance" because of sustained criticism of the programme's ethical
basis.[10] Research on germ line treatment and somatic cell treatment
was deleted from the programme. The future guidelines will probably
be rather restrictive. The parliamentary assembly of the Council of
Europe endorses a "right to a genetic inheritance which has not been
artificially interfered with" as a basic human right in its recommendation 934(1982) and proposes the establishment of a list of severe
diseases for which genetic treatment is warranted.

## Confidentiality of medical records

The rules concerning access to medical records vary in the different
member states. In some countries patients have a right to access, in
others the records are the exclusive property of doctors. The
discussion in the official European bodies has mainly concentrated on
securing confidentiality when new technology is used. The Council of
Ministers is preparing a general directive concerned with confidentiality of personal information but this directive is still under negotiation. The Council of Europe has issued a recommendation on the
impact of new technologies on health services, which states that
protection of confidentiality must be secured in all systems.

---

### Useful addresses and journals

The Commission of the EC, the European Parliament, and the
Council of Europe have information offices in all member states and can
supply copies of the relevant documents.

European Association of Centers of Medical Ethics, Promenade de
l'Alma 51, B-1200 Brussels, Belgium.

The European Society for the Philosophy of Medicine and Health
Care, Secretary, Professor Dr Henk ten Have, Department of Ethics,
Philosophy and History of Medicine, Catholic University of Nijmegan,
Verlengde Groenestraat 75, PO Box 9101, 6500 HB Nijmegen, Nether-
lands.

The Standing Committee of Doctors of the EC, Ordem dos Médicos,
Av Almirante Gago Coutinho 151, 1700 Lisbon, Portugal.

*The Bulletin of Medical Ethics, The Journal of Medical Ethics, Medicine
and Ethics* and the *International Digest of Health Legislation* cover
developments in European medical ethics and law.

---

# Testing for HIV

The Council of Ministers of the EC,[11][12] the committee of ministers of the Council of Europe, the general assembly of the World Health Organisation, and the Standing Committee of Doctors of the EC have issued statements on AIDS that underline the importance of voluntary testing and strict confidentiality. They emphasise that any discrimination against people who are HIV positive is an unacceptable infringement of human rights.

It is, however, difficult to ensure full confidentiality when access to testing for HIV becomes more widespread. In Denmark a private firm has already advertised a do it yourself test. They send out a blood collecting device and analyse the blood sent back. The amount of blood needed is small and there is no way of checking that the person requesting the test is the person whose blood is being tested.

## Organ donation

Organ donation systems also differ. Most countries have an opting in system where donors have to state their willingness to donate, but some countries—Belgium is one—have an opting out system where consent for donation is presumed if there is no contravening statement from the deceased.[13] In recent WHO guidelines on transplantation both systems are described but no specific system is recommended. A common policy would be preferable to increase efficiency in procuring, distributing, and using organs, but the exact design of the system will probably cause a lot of discussion.

The general assembly of the WHO twice unanimously issued resolutions calling for the prohibition of trade in human organs, and the Council of Europe has issued a similar recommendation. Most European legislatures have enacted laws to this effect, but a few countries, such as Ireland and Netherlands, lack any legislation on organ donation.

## Euthanasia and assisted suicide

Anyone working in medicine knows that euthanasia is practised even though it is prohibited in all European countries. It may well be called something else, but there is no doubt that the main purpose is to hasten the process of dying. The practice is publicly acknowledged in Netherlands, although it is not legal. It is estimated that 1·8% of all deaths in Netherlands are caused by the intentional administration of lethal drugs.[15] A Dutch member of the European parliament has proposed a resolution on the care of the terminally ill, which urges the commission to work for the introduction of voluntary euthanasia.[15] This proposal is still under consideration. The legalisation of euthanasia has been rejected by the Standing Committee of Doctors of the EC in its declaration on euthanasia adopted in 1987 and by the World Medical Association in its declaration adopted at the 39th world medical assembly in Madrid in 1987.

## The way forward

The problems that will face doctors in the EC in the future are manifold, but two will give rise to ethical debates: changes in the relationship between doctors and patients, and problems with the just allocation of resources.

Patients will want to be more involved in the decisions about their treatment. They will want to be better informed, but they will still want to be able to lay the final responsibility for the decisions on their doctor. These seemingly incompatible demands must be incorporated in a new conception of the doctor-patient relationship. The main challenge for doctors will be to resist the intrusion of legal mechanisms without resisting the necessary changes in the relationship. Doctors will have to learn new ways of interacting with their patients. It may be that what patients want is not the emphasis on patient autonomy to the exclusion of all other values which has dominated the American scene. If cooperation, kindness, and friendship are allowed a role a good relationship is more likely to develop.

The allocation of health care resources will also become more pressing in the new Europe. The discussion in Britain about the differences between the poor north and the affluent south east is just a prelude to the European discussion about these problems. The social and regional differences highlighted in the Black report pale in comparison to the differences between the European regions.[16] And the differences in the present EC will be greatly expanded if and when the new democracies in eastern Europe are allowed to join.

The committee of ministers of the Council of Europe has issued a recommendation on making medical care universally available, which specifies a wide range of health care that should be available to every citizen as a right. This ideal is not yet fulfilled in the poor regions of Europe, but the medical profession must actively work to achieve it.

These challenges must be met individually, nationally, and at the European level. But it will not be an easy task. Not only are there cultural differences but the climate to discuss these issues varies between the member states. It is not possible to discuss freely euthanasia, prenatal screening, or abortion in all states. The European Society for the Philosophy of Medicine and Health Care (a neutral academic society) had to move its 1990 meeting from Germany to the Netherlands because of threats of disruption.

So unless we aim for the lowest common denominator we may find it much more dfficult to reach a common ethical policy than a common defence policy or a common monetary policy.

1 Office for Official Publications of the European Communities. *1992—the social dimension*. Luxemburg: Office for Official Publications of the European Communities, 1990.
2 Holm S. New Danish law: human life begins at conception. *J Med Ethics* 1988;**14**:77-8.
3 Isambert F-A. Ethics committes in France. *J Med Philos* 1989;**14**:445-56.
4 Walters L. Commissions and bioethics. *J Med Philos* 1989;**14**:363-8.
5 Glover J. *Fertility and the family: the Glover report on reproductive technologies to the European commission*. London: Fourth Estate, 1989.
6 Congregation for the Doctrine of Faith. *Instruction on respect for human life in its origin and on the dignity of procreation*. Vatican: Congregation for the Doctrine of Faith, 1987.
7 Council of Europe. *Human artificial procreation*. Strasburg: Council of Europe, 1989.
8 Kasimba P. A summary of legislation relating to IVF. In: Singer P, Kuhse H, Buckle S, Dawson K, Kasimba P, eds. *Embryo experimentation*. Sydney: Cambridge University Press, 1990: 227-36.
9 European Science Foundation. *Report on genome research 1991*. Southampton: European Science Foundation, 1991.
10 Rix BA. Should ethical concerns regulate science? The European experience with the human genome project. *Bioethics* 1991;**5**:250-6.
11 Conclusions of the council and the ministers for health, meeting within the council, on 16 May 1989 on AIDS. *Official Journal of the European Communities No C* 1989 July 22:185/4-6.
12 Conclusions of the council and of the ministers for health, meeting within the council, of 3 December 1990 on AIDS. *Official Journal of the European Communities No C* 1990 December 12: 329/21-2.
13 Binamé G. Organ transplantation: a chronicle of a long-awaited law. *International Digest of Health Legislation* 1990;**41**:336-9.
14 Van der Maas PJ, van Delden JJM, Pijnenborg L, Looman CWN. Euthanasia and other medical decisions concerning the end of life. *Lancet* 1991;ii: 669-74.
15 Anonymous. European support for euthanasia? *Bull Med Eth* 1991;**69**:25-7.
16 Department of Health and Social Security. *Inequalities in health: report of a research working group*. London: DHSS, 1980. (Black report.)

# European law, medicine, and the social charter

CHRIS HUGHES

In 1974 Lord Denning said that the Treaty of Rome "is like an inrushing tide. . . . It flows into the estuaries and up the rivers. It cannot be held back."[1] He was confirming what had been apparent from the treaty: "If the Court of Justice finds that a member state has failed to fulfil an obligation under this treaty, the state shall be required to take the necessary measures to comply with the judgment of the Court of Justice." So in matters of law parliament would no longer have the last word and in many areas the law would be made by the European institutions and determined in accordance with the decisions of the European Court.

But the doctrine of the sovereignty of parliament has been a long time dying because of judicial conservatism and political prevarication. A contemporary commentator wrote of the European Communities Act 1972, "This unique act is a fascinating exercise in equivocation, a wilful manifestation of legislative schizophrenia . . . the United Kingdom government has seated parliament on two horses, one straining towards the preservation of parliamentary sovereignty, the other galloping in the general direction of community law supremacy."[2]

There is a time limit for European legislation to be translated into the law of member states. This has given rise to confusion over the interpretation of United Kingdom legislation, which a grudging government has passed in supposed compliance with European Community (EC) law. In addition to trying to resolve conflicts between the EC regulation and the United Kingdom law, British courts have had difficulty simply understanding the regulation. As Lord Diplock said in one leading case, "The European court, in

124

contrast to English courts, applies teleological rather than historical methods to the interpretation of the treaties and other community legislation. It seeks to give effect to what it conceives to be the spirit rather than the letter of the treaties; sometimes, indeed, to an English judge, it may seem to the exclusion of the letter."[3]

The conflict over parliamentary sovereignty recently came to a head in the Factortame case.[4] In a long running conflict over fishing quotas parliament passed the Merchant Shipping Act 1988, which prevented foreign owned vessels registering in Britain and getting access to British quotas. Spanish owners applied to the British courts, which in turn sought a preliminary ruling from the European court. This held that British courts had power temporarily to suspend the operation of the act pending determination of whether it conflicted with European law.[5]

In an even more recent case the European court held that the relevant directive did not create obligations which could be relied upon by one private individual against another.[6] A national court was, however, bound to interpret national law in accordance with the terms of the directive. It therefore had to disapply a provision in national law to secure compliance with the terms of the directive since the directive constituted an exhaustive statement of the relevant law even though it had not been implemented in the member state.

This decision seemed to sweep away much of the confusion, that had surrounded British equal pay cases. In one case the plaintiff succeeded because she was a public employee while another failed

---

**Conflicting issues**

The European Commission and the United Kingdom government are in conflict over the following commission proposals[7]:
- Protection for pregnant and nursing mothers from being obliged to work shifts
- Fourteen weeks' maternity leave on full pay
- Equal rights for part time and temporary staff to pensions, holidays, training, and rights in redundancy
- Minimum wage
- Rights of workers to participate in employer decisions
- Action to assist disabled people
- Greater protection for employees threatened with collective dismissal
- Controls on hours of work

because she was not. Now it seemed clear that the courts could rely equally on the provisions of European legislation whether directly enacted in the United Kingdom or not. Even if parliament passed a law in direct contravention of the European legislation any right in European law would be enforceable through any relevant British court. In several recent cases in England, however, the Court of Appeal has ruled: "... does not in my opinion enable or constrain a British court to distort the meaning of a British statute in order to enforce against an individual a community directive which has no direct effect between individuals."[6] Until such a case goes to the House of Lords and the opinion of the European court is sought this confusion will remain.

## Single market and qualified majority voting

The European treaty was revised in 1986 to enable the community to accelerate the process of integration. It sacrificed the de facto right to a veto and introduced qualified majority voting in the Council of Ministers on measures necessary to achieve this end. A total of 76 votes are split between the 12 members, each member having from 10 (United Kingdom, France, Germany, and Italy) to two (Luxemburg). Fifty four votes are needed to carry a proposal. The

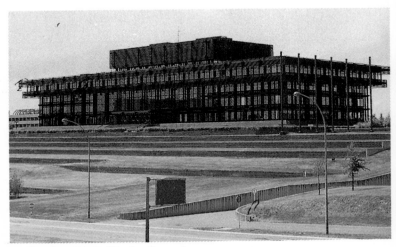

The European Court of Justice, Luxemburg

European Commission has been criticised by Britain for "dressing up" measures advancing the social dimension of Europe as part of the single market and bringing them within the qualified majority procedure. Even where majority voting is available the Council of Europe prefers to move by consensus.

## Maastricht

The public relations explosion surrounding the meeting in Maastricht in December 1991 obscured the deep confusion of the participants about the consequences and importance of their actions. The British government's deep seated objections to the commission's social action programme led to Britain not adhering to the social charter 1989. At Maastricht the United Kingdom insisted that the social chapter proposed for the Political Union Treaty (due for ratification by all 12 states in 1992 and taking effect in 1993) should not be included. Instead it was incorporated as a protocol to enable the other 11 members to proceed with the social charter proposals.[7]

Nevertheless, work on all social charter proposals will proceed initially on the basis of seeking agreement among the 12; if that is impossible then consensus among the 11 will be sought. The agreements made under the protocol will be taken within the framework of the EC's institutions "on loan" to the signatory states. This is clearly an unstable position. The European court has already ruled that the draft agreement on a European economic area which would bring into effect a close association between the EC and the countries of EFTA threatened the autonomy of the community's legal order and was incompatible with the Treaty of Rome. There will probably be similar difficulties with the proposed protocol. Arguments are being advanced in the European Parliament that since the United Kingdom will not be bound by the proposals its members in the European Parliament should take no part in the discussions.

In the meantime the government continues to oppose many of the key proposed directives that are seen by the commission as essential to maintain broad support for the "ever closer union." The commission's objective is a core of social rights applicable throughout the community. The lack of consensus in the Council of Ministers is likely to mean, at most, amendments to social and employment legislation rather than the coherent framework of rights proposed until the protocol is implemented.

Under a protocol to the economic and monetary union provisions of

127

the treaty, the United Kingdom will be able to opt out of the move to full monetary union based on a single currency. This will come into effect between 1 January 1997 and 1 January 1999; Britain would have to exercise its option in the middle of the decade.

## Health and safety

The community adopted a framework directive on health and safety in 1989 and is now adopting specific measures requiring national implementation by the end of 1992. The measures contain a healthy dose of worker participation, training, and rights of consultation as well as requirements with respect to health surveillance. The requirement that "particularly sensitive groups must be protected against dangers which specifically affect them" seems to make the offer of hepatitis B virus inoculation to many health staff mandatory and could have implications for the availability of prophylactic ziduvodine after needlestick injury.

Much of the specific provision makes explicit what was implicit in the Health and Safety at Work Act 1974. Among the directives already adopted are ones on the manual lifting of heavy loads; use of work equipment; carcinogens; safety clothing; and visual display units, which will require free eye tests and breaks from the use of the equipment. The last directive, 90/679 (national implementation by 26 November 1993), is intended to protect workers from exposure to biological agents at work. It requires regular risk assessment in accordance with a statutory classification scheme, and where risk exists exposure must be prevented or kept as low as possible. Records of exposures are required to be kept for up to 40 years.

One key health and safety proposal still under consideration would make manadatory daily rest periods of 12 hours, at least one day off a week, normal hours for night workers not to exceed an average of eight hours a shift, and prohibiting overtime for night workers in occupations involving special hazards or heavy physical or mental strain. The British government is known to be unhappy with this proposal, especially with respect to its impact on the NHS, and it is unlikely to be adopted except under the Maastricht protocol.

## Health

One principle of EC law, subsidiarity, requires that the EC should not undertake tasks more suitable for national governments. Health

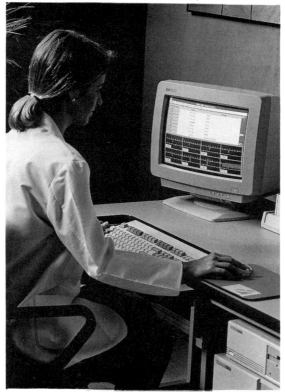

Specific EC measures on health and safety require work
breaks and free eye tests for users of visual display units

care is recognised as one such area and it is unlikely that there will be
any uniformity of provision of health care in Europe. Nevertheless,
the impact of European law is profound and pervasive and directly
affects many facets of medicine. Article 51 of the Treaty of Rome
provides that the community shall "adopt such measures in the field of
social security as are necessary to provide freedom of movement for
workers." The purpose is as far as possible to abolish territorial
limitations on the application of the different social security schemes.
This supplements national schemes to ensure that a migrant worker is
not disadvantaged by moving within the community. Regulations
made under the article cover a broad expanse of benefits, including
reimbursement of expenses for medical treatment, medicines, and

nursing. In particular there is a right for people entitled to benefits in one member state to receive treatment in another at the expense of their own state if they obtain prior approval. There are restrictions on refusal of approval, in particular where there is some degree of urgency in obtaining treatment.

In two cases, Mrs G Pierik, a Dutch midwife on invalidity benefit, successfully challenged a refusal by the Netherlands to provide her with spa treatment in Germany.[8] The regulations were held to apply to pensioners seeking any appropriate treatment even if it is not usually provided at home. In both cases the British government submitted arguments to the European court which would have had the effect of restricting the right to seek treatment. The system for administering this right in Britain (form E112) does not seem to be designed to encourage the exercise of this right. About 125 applications were approved in 1990; many more were rejected. The Department of Health clearly views the procedure as appropriate only in exceptional cases, and there is a strong reluctance to countenance it as a means of accelerating treatment, despite the obligation to take account of the current state of the patient's health and the likely course of the disease. As with the reluctance of health authorities to make large budgetary provision for extracontractual referrals, the department sees no reason to spend money in other European countries which it is not prepared to spend in Britain. Whether this reluctance is in accordance with the current law is debatable. These regulations are to be extended to self employed people and their families.

In pursing an internal market for the NHS the government has sought to ensure that the market remains a British market. The NHS and Community Care Act provides for NHS contracts to be between specific NHS bodies and not to be enforceable in the courts. It is anticipated, however, that NHS bodies will enter into similar contracts with the private sector. In that case article 59, which establishes the freedom to provide services across frontiers, seems to apply, certainly where contracts are being considered with the private sector and possibly NHS contracts as well.

## Sex discrimination

A series of decisions of the European court have exposed the inadequacies of British law in relation to discrimination on the grounds of sex and required the government to bring forward the Sex Discrimination Act 1986. Barber held that discrimination on the grounds

---

**Data protection**

The European Commission is proposing sweeping extensions to existing legislation protecting personal data including:
- Application to manual as well as computer files
- Duty of private sector processors to notify data subjects of their activities and the subject's right to ban such data processing
- Right to knowledge of and access to public sector files on the subject of the data
- A ban, except in cases of important public interest, to the automatic processing of data on racial or ethnic origin; political, religious or philosophical views; health; or sexual activities without the written consent of the subject of the data

---

of sex in occupational pension schemes was contrary to article 119 of the treaty (equal pay).[9] This is having a profound effect on the pensions market. In particular the decision that article 119 may not be relied on for claiming entitlement to a pension with effect before the date of judgment has created confusion. The extent to which the right to backdated or future benefits exists may be clarified in litigation related to the Coloroll pension scheme, which has been referred to the European Court, and also by possible European legislation.

In 1990 the Court of Appeal decided that different age limits governing eligibility for severe disablement and invalid care allowances were not a necessary consequence of the difference in retirement age and were unlawful. But in proceedings brought by the Equal Opportunities Commission the divisional court has upheld the view of the secretary of state for social security that the minimum hours requirement for unfair dismissal rights, though indirectly discriminatory on the grounds of sex, was justifiable. This case will be the subject of appeal.[10]

## Nationality and immigration

Article 48 of the Treaty of Rome provides for the abolition of discrimination based on nationality in employment between workers of member states, and article 58 provides for the right to pursue activities on a self employed basis. Although regulations providing for mutual recognition of medical qualifications have been in place for some years, the General Medical Council has registered only 6500 EC doctors and new registrations are running at approximately 1000 a year. It is believed that most remain for a relatively short period. The number of British doctors working in the rest of the EC is believed to be small. One problem remains: the directive currently regulating movement of doctors provides for the mutual recognition of EC qualifications of EC citizens. It discriminates against holders of non-EC qualifications who are EC citizens and non-EC nationals who hold EC qualifications. At Maastricht it was agreed to move towards cooperation on immigration and asylum policies. Explicit reference was made to respect the European Convention on Human Rights and the Convention on the Status of Refugees. In a statement condemning the increase in racism and xenophobia the Council of Europe called for steps to be taken at national and community level to combat discrimination and xenophobia and to strengthen the legal protection of third country nationals in all members states.

## Medical accident litigation

The wide range of arrangements for the delivery of health care is mirrored by the variation in the law relating to medical negligence and the differences in insurance arrangements. While the basic analysis of negligence is the same, the burdens of proof vary. The community is considering legislation that would impose a uniform code of liability for the providers of defective services.

EC studies indicate that while in the United Kingdom and Italy the burden is on the plaintiff to show negligence, in Spain, Denmark, Greece, and Belgium the burden of proof is reversed and in Germany the doctrine of the positive isolation of contractual duty has a similar effect. Furthermore, in Germany instead of the plaintiff proving that the defendant's negligence caused the damage the concept of the "sphere of risk"—that is, the factors within the control of the defendant —effectively reverses the burden in many cases. The insurance arrangements across the community are similarly diverse, with insurance being mandatory in all forms of practice in Germany, voluntary in Portugal, and mandatory or voluntary depending on the nature of the practice in Italy.

The European Commission argues that this wide variation in the substantive law has the effect of inhibiting the free market in services across Europe and has proposed legislation that would reverse the burden of proof of negligence in cases where physical damage has been caused by the defective provision of services. The proposal follows on from the directive on defective products which was the basis of the Consumer Protection Act 1987 and its introduction of the concept of a product being defective if it is not as safe as "persons generally are entitled to expect." An initial proposal for the implementation of a system of no fault liability was dropped after pressure from interest groups and because of a reluctance to take such a radical step. It seems unlikely that such a proposal will re-emerge. The wide implications of the proposals have had increasing exposure, and as a result of criticism it seems likely that there will be a separate directive dealing with the defective provision of health care. Any legislation is likely to be based on the principle of reversing the burden of proof, but it is unlikely that there will be a move towards a Swedish no fault system.

The impact of such a directive on medical negligence litigation is uncertain. It could raise expectations of the possibility of compensation and thus contribute to an American style growth in such litigation, which has been a feature of the past decade. But although the burden is shifted, this is effective only in the absence of contrary evidence. In a civil case the burden of proof is on a balance of probabilities—that is, a fact, inference, or causal relationship is proved if it is established as having a probability of more than a half. In practice a contested case will still see the serried ranks of expert witnesses giving evidence as to what is and is not acceptable to a respectable body of medical opinion, especially since "the mere fact that a better service existed will not constitute a fault." Since the draft embodies more restrictive time limits to bring proceedings than are presently applicable there would be two classes of proceedings: those under the directive and those brought in common law. The draft directive, if enacted, would be unlikely to resolve the problems of delay, legal costs, uncertainty, and disruption inherent in the present system of medical negligence litigation.

## Conclusion

Over the past 19 years, although many politicians have treated the community as an external body concerned purely with economic policy, the United Kingdom has acquired a written constitution and seen many important changes to its law and the rights of its citizens — to the confusion of politician, citizen, and lawyer alike. The changes are continuing at an accelerating pace, and the reluctance of politicians to comprehend that political power follows economic influence has caused Britain to adopt a policy in negotiations that has caused political isolation in the community and is untenable.

1  Bulmer (HP) *v* J Bollinger SA [1974]. 2 All ER 1226.
2  De Smith SA. *Constitutional and administrative law*. 2nd ed. London: Penguin, 1973.
3  Henn and Darby *v* DPP [1980] 2 All ER 166.
4  Factortame Ltd *v* Secretary of State for Transport (No 2) [1991] 1 All ER 70.
5  Marleasing SA *v* La Comercial Internacional de Alimentacion SA. European Court, case 106/89.
6  Webb *v* Emo Air Cargo (UK) Ltd [1992] All ER 43.
7  European Commission. *First report on the application of the European community's social charter*. Brussels: European Commission, 1992.
8  Bestuur van het Algemeen Ziekenfonds Drenthe-Platteland *v* Pierik. European Court, cases 117/77 and 182/78.
9  Barber *v* Guardian Royal Exchange Assurance Group [1990] 19 IRLR 240.
10  R *v* Secretary of State for Employment ex p Equal Opportunities Commission [1991] 20 IRLR 493.

# Equal opportunities: progress so far

PETER FORSTER

According to Docksey, "equality policy is one of the few relatively successful and advanced employment policies at community level."[1] Indeed, gender equality is enshrined in article 119 of the Treaty of Rome. But despite a considerable number of initiatives and the substantial increase of women in the labour force, the European Commission reported in 1989 that progress in achieving equality has been slow, with women remaining largely confined to traditional occupations, relatively low level jobs, and atypical forms of work which do not provide the same levels of protection and benefits as traditional types of work.[2]

## Coordinating unit

In the European Community equal opportunity matters are coordinated by the commission's equal opportunities unit in directorate general V, which ensures the application of directives and draft proposals, encourages positive action, and monitors the application of action programmes. It also runs a women's information service, which produces regular information bulletins and runs seminars.

The problem is that, though aimed at achieving equality between the sexes, most of the initiatives and policies adopted at an EC level deal mainly with the unequal treatment of women at the workplace—for example, dismissal, maintenance of rights in pregnancy, and training.

The commitment to equal opportunities enshrined in the Treaty of Rome has been extended by five equality directives and agreed by all member states, and despite protestations by Britain the directives

---

**Women in Europe**

Women account for over one third of the western European workforce and just under one third of the medical workforce, yet the participation of women is below that in the United States and eastern Europe. There are still 21 million women between the ages of 25 and 49 "economically inactive" in the community, and average pay is still only 80% of the average pay for men.

In the United Kingdom women make up a higher proportion of the workforce than in any other EC country, except Denmark, but the earnings gap is wider than in any other country. On average, full time women workers in Britain earn 77% of the earnings of men. They fare worse in terms of maternity rights, access to child care— there are places available for only 2% of under 5s at state and private nurseries combined — training opportunities, and promotion to senior positions.[5]

---

have been incorporated into national laws as part of an EC wide social action programme.

*The equal pay directive* sought to "facilitate the practical application of the principle of equality" as outlined in the Treaty of Rome. It included the idea that equal pay should apply to work of "equal value" and not just to identical work. The obligations imposed on the United Kingdom by the directive are included in the Equal Pay (Amendment) Regulations 1983.

*The equal treatment directive* of 1976 provided for the equal treatment of men and women in conditions and in access to employment, vocational training, and promotion. The directive prohibited all gender based discrimination at work, both direct and indirect. In the United Kingdom the Employment Act 1989 amended the sex discrimination legislation and statutory redundancy scheme in order to comply with the directive.

*The first social security directive* of 1986 established the right to equal treatment in both statutory and supplementary social security schemes.

*The second social security directive* of 1986 implemented the principle of equal treatment for men and women in occupational social security schemes (covering employed and self employed people). The directive allowed for the deferment of the equalisation of pension age and survivors' benefits until statutory equalisation was achieved. This is being considered by the United Kingdom government.

*The self employed directive* of 1986 aimed to extend protection against sex discrimination to all self employed people as well as to those whose employment status was unclear. It covers financial support for established business, social security, and temporary replacement services during maternity.

## Equal opportunities action programmes

The first equal opportunities action programme, which covered the period 1982-5, set out to ensure the observance of the principle of equal treatment by the development of community legal action and to promote equal opportunity in practice through positive action programmes.

The second equal opportunities action programme (1986-90) aimed to consolidate steps already taken so that "equal opportunities become an accepted part of everyday life for all community citizens." Seven areas were specifically targeted:
- Improved application of existing equal treatment provisions
- Education and training
- Employment (including more positive action programmes)
- New technology
- Social protection and social security
- Sharing of family and occupational responsibility through awareness raising, child care facilities, and flexibility of working patterns
- Changing traditional male and female attitudes.

Progress under this programme has included legal measures in the form of draft directives proposing, among other things, the equalisation of retirement ages and ending the discrimination in pension rights against women who have interrupted their employment. Another important directive which failed to be adopted (on account of the United Kingdom veto) proposed shifting the burden of proof in equal treatment cases to the employer—that is, discrimination would be presumed until the employer could prove otherwise.

The commission's third equal opportunities action programme, launched in 1991, covers the period 1991-5 and seeks to "promote women's full participation in, and to revalue their contribution to economic and social life." The programme covers proposals on the financing of child care facilities, the adoption of a recommendation on child care services, and a code of good conduct on the protection of pregnancy and maternity.

137

## Positive action programme

The legislative initiatives have been underpinned by a positive action programme started in 1984 to "promote a better balance between the sexes in employment, eliminate the idea of a traditional division of roles in society between men and women, encourage participation of women in sectors where they are underrepresented and at high levels of responsibility."

The programme is implemented by means of a recommendation rather than a directive, and although it does not have to be incorported into national law, it is expected that all member states will respond to it in practical terms. So far the only EC member states to give legal and financial backing to the programme have been Belgium, Italy, and Netherlands.

Since 1990 Belgium has had a compulsory positive action programme for public sector employees plus voluntary programmes for the private sector, with financial and practical backing via specially

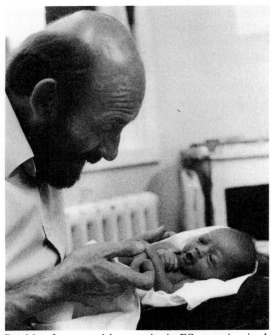

Provision for parental leave varies in EC countries; in the United Kingdom there is no legal right to parental leave

seconded civil servants. Netherlands has a policy of partially subsidising child care costs for working parents as well as a compulsory positive action programme in the civil service. In 1991 Italy passed its first positive action programme together with legal and financial backing. In Germany two regions have programmes for the public sector, while Spain, Denmark, and Greece have national plans of action for equal treatment of men and women. This year the Republic of Ireland has published a report by a commission on the status of women.

## Parental leave

In its 1989 social action programme, which accompanied the social charter, the European Commission proposed the adoption of a draft directive on parental leave and leave for family reasons. At present there is a wide disparity among EC member states on leave available to both the mother and father—generous in Denmark, Italy, and France; poor in Ireland, Netherlands, and the United Kingdom (the country with no legal right to parental leave). The directive proposed a minimum of three months' full time leave for each parent within two years of the birth or adoption of a child. The leave could be paid or unpaid but if paid the cost should be met by the state rather than the employer. This measure requires unanimity for adoption and is unlikely—given the United Kingdom's opposition—to make much headway at present.

## Pregnancy

The Single European Act 1986 added articles 100A and 118A to the Treaty of Rome. This allowed the European institutions to sidestep the national veto, particularly the United Kingdom's. Article 118, which deals largely with health and safety at work issues, was used by the commission to advance a draft directive on the protection of pregnant women at work. The draft directive includes:
● Measures to ensure the protection of pregnant and breastfeeding women against exposure to harmful agents and processes
● Measures requiring the reorganisation of the working conditions and hours of pregnant and nursing employees without "material disadvantage to them"
● The right to a substantial period of paid maternity leave
● The prohibition of dismissal on pregnancy grounds.

> ### Underrepresentation in medicine
>
> The NHS, which has 1·1 million employees—75% of whom are women—reflects the general position in the United Kingdom. Women are unequally represented in the different occupational groups. Isabel Allen showed that while in general women medical students were "more strongly motivated than men towards a medical career" and made good progress through medical school, house officer, and senior house officer grades, they progressed far less quickly than their male counterparts at registrar level and above.[6]
>
> A recent study of women doctors and their careers showed that although almost equal numbers of men and women students qualify from medical school, women hold only 15% of consultant posts, only 3% of consultant posts in surgical specialties, and represent 1% of general surgeons, while they are overrepresented in the lower training grades.[7]

These proposals require only a qualified majority for adoption by the Council of Europe.

Under existing United Kingdom legislation dealing with sex discrimination the treatment of pregnant women at work has to be compared with the treatment or expected treatment of a "comparable" male employee or partner. The European Court of Justice in the Dekker case decided that as pregnancy was a uniquely feminine condition any detriment suffered by a woman because of pregnancy was directly discriminatory.[3] One of the many implications of this judgment for British employers is that the "comparable male" approach may no longer be good law. Lawyers are still untangling the legal threads of this decision, but it will no doubt be a cause célèbre in the quest for equality in the workplace.*

## United Kingdom response

The United Kingdom has been reluctant to legislate on equality issues. Opportunity 2000, which was launched by John Major in 1991, was a voluntary scheme without legal or financial teeth aimed at improving prospects for women in the United Kingdom. Prompted

---

* In the first of the Dekker judgment in the United Kingdom (Webb v EMO Air Cargo (UK) Ltd) the Court of Appeal upheld the "comparable male" approach. Nevertheless, the possibility remains for industrial tribunals in future cases to follow the constitutional and interpretative decisions of the European Court of Justice in preference to those of the Court of Appeal or the House of Lords.

by the charity Business in the Community, 14 of Britain's top employers—including the NHS—have set out their own 10 year targets to improve the position of women. As a signatory to Opportunity 2000 the NHS Management Executive commissioned a report from the Office for Public Management to profile the "issues relating to the role of women in the NHS and to build on progress in providing equal opportunities for women."[4]

The report identified four general and pervasive barriers to equality: outmoded attitudes about the role of women; direct and indirect discrimination; the absence of proper child care provision; and inflexible structures for work and careers. It noted that discrimination could take many forms but was particularly apparent in subjective and informal selection procedures; stereotyped assumptions about the ability, character, suitability, and natural role of women; the use of insider, word of mouth, and old boys' networks; unnecessary age bars; and excessive mobility requirements.

## Conclusion

Although the cause of equality enjoys a general measure of acceptance throughout the community, progress has been slow. As the commission's third action programme implies, perhaps the time is right to "pause and consider" what steps should be taken to increase public awareness of the law on equality, to monitor developments in member states, and develop a system for spreading information and legal standards in what is a most complex field.

1 Docksey C. The principle of equality between women and men as a fudamental right under community law. *Industrial Law Journal* 1991;4:258.
2 European Commission. *First annual report on employment in Europe.* Brussels: European Commission, 1989.
3 Dekker *v* Stichting Vormings-Centrum voor Junge Volwassen (VJV-Centrum) plus (1991). Case 177/88.
4 NHS Management Executive. *Equal opportunities for women in the NHS.* London: Department of Health, 1991.
5 Equal Opportunities Commission. *Women and men in Britain.* London: Equal Opportunities Commission, 1991.
6 Allen I. *Discussing doctors' careers.* London: Policy Studies Institute, 1989.
7 Joint Working Party. *Women doctors and their careers.* London: Department of Health, 1991.

# The way ahead

CHRIS HAM, PHILIP BERMAN

European health policy stands at the crossroads. The agreement reached by members of the European Community at Maastricht in December includes a new chapter on public health to be incorporated in the Treaty of Rome. Whereas previous health initiatives developed in the European Community in an ad hoc way from a fragile legal base,[1] in future there will be a specific mandate for action. As a consequence, the community's influence on health policy is likely to increase, particularly in relation to public health.

The wording of the new chapter indicates that the main priority will be given to disease prevention and health promotion. Its aim is to tackle "major health scourges" through research and health education. This will probably mean extending previous initiatives on cancer, AIDS, and drug misuse. In addition, the chapter emphasises that "health protection demands shall form a constituent part of the community's other policies," which opens up the prospect of taking action on policies in related areas, such as the environment and agricultural policy, which affect health. This would make it difficult to justify subsidies to tobacco growers that far outweigh the resources devoted to combating cancer.[2]

European health ministers, including William Waldegrave,[3] have taken pains to point out that no attempt will be made to harmonise the financing and provision of health services. Here the community principle of subsidiarity operates[4]; these issues are regarded as better handled by national and regional governments. Any move to establish health services on a common basis would be firmly resisted at this stage, although in the longer term pressures may well emerge to reduce differences between national systems.

142

These pressures are most likely to arise through completion of the single market. The greater mobility of people accompanying the development of a single market will make more transparent the variations that exist among member states.[5] Not only will this test the strength of the community's procedures for dealing with the provision of health care to citizens of one state who work or live in another but it could also lead to demands for convergence in the provision of services. Those responsible for policies relating to social protection in the European Commission are already beginning to think through these issues, and over time greater comparability of entitlements and standards between countries may result.[6]

Regardless of any official initiatives the 1990s are likely to see more medical tourism. Patients from southern states such as Italy and Greece will travel in greater numbers than previously to centres of excellence elsewhere in the community. Equally, people who live in border areas with good transport links may opt for medical treatment in states other than where they live.

Purchasers and providers of health care are already operating across national frontiers. For example, a Danish hospital flies 30 patients each week to its hospital in Malaga for recuperation at a cost (including airfare) substantially lower than that for similar treatment in Denmark. The largest German private health insurance company has opened offices in Belgium, Netherlands, Spain, France, and the United Kingdom. Closer to home, private insurers in Britain are beginning to offer subscribers the option of treatment outside the United Kingdom, and a group of NHS managers are seeking to market their services in Europe.

In parallel with patient mobility, closer European integration may result in greater movement of health care professionals. To date this has been limited, even though the European Community has promoted mutual recognition of qualifications. Language and cultural differences undoubtedly inhibit extensive interchanges, although staff shortages and surpluses in different countries may encourage greater mobility than in the past. If this were to happen it might force the community to take a closer interest in manpower planning and distribution to ensure an adequate supply of properly trained professionals in different countries.

As these comments indicate, much uncertainty remains about the future. Nevertheless, one thing is clear: the new chapter on public health provides a basis for more concerted action than in the past, and an opportunity now exists to develop cooperation between member states to tackle the principal causes of morbidity and death in Europe.

Because of the vague wording of the chapter, almost everything hinges on interpretation in practice. Of particular interest is the commitment to use "incentive measures" to ensure a high level of health protection. This is a new phrase in the vocabulary of the community, and it indicates that public health policy will not be characterised by the directives and regulations that have legal force in other areas of European policy. Instead alternative approaches will be emphasised, the nature of which have yet to be specified. In this respect, as in the definition of public health to be adopted by the commission, there is much to play for.

Now is therefore the time for interested parties to mobilise to help shape European public health policy. The commission itself has only a small staff working on this topic, and it relies heavily on advice from experts and professional associations. Although the Standing Committee of Doctors in the European Community has found it difficult to exert influence in the past,[7] the British Medical Association has recently committed resources to strengthening the work of the standing committee. Other organisations are also getting their act together, as the recent establishment of the European Public Health Alliance indicates. Although attention is likely to be focused on the public health chapter, other areas of policy should not be ignored. Health services may well be affected by generic European legislation (as in relation to the liability of suppliers for negligence[4]), and those working in the health sector will need alerting to the implications of innocuous sounding directives emanating from the community.

Apart from seeking to influence Brussels, recognising the need to work through national governments is also important. In England the Department of Health has recently reorganised its international division to give more emphasis to European Community activities, and it is vital that the work of the division feeds directly into the mainstream of NHS management. In the second half of the year the British government holds the presidency of the community, which creates an opportunity for it to exercise leadership in the development of European policy. There is talk of a public health initiative to coincide with the presidency, and this would set the direction for the future. With *The Health Of The Nation* providing the framework for action in England[8] an initiative to establish a strategy on the health of the community would be an imaginative way for the government to demonstrate the possibilities contained in the new public health chapter.

1 Smith R. European research: back to pre-eminence? *BMJ* 1992;**304**:899-903.
1a Richards T. 1992 and all that. *BMJ* 1991;**303**:1319-22.
2 Bosanquet N. Europe and tobacco. *BMJ* 1992;**304**:370-2.
3 Waldegrave W. The health of Europe. *BMJ* 1992;**304**:370-2.
4 Hughes C. European law, medicine, and the social charter. *BMJ* 1992;**304**:700-2.
5 Stallnecht K. Nursing in Europe. *BMJ* 1992;**304**:561-2.
6 Schneider M, Dennerlein RK, Kose A, Scholtes L. *Health care baskets*. Augsburg: BASYS, 1991.
7 Richards T. Who speaks for whom? *BMJ* 1992;**304**:103-6.
8 Secretary of State for Health. *The health of the nation*. London: HMSO, 1991.

# Index